Low-Fat Lies

Low-Fat Lies

*High-Fat Frauds and the
Healthiest Diet in the World*

Kevin Vigilante, M.D., M.P.H.,
and Mary Flynn, Ph.D.

LifeLine
Press

A Regnery Publishing Company • Washington, DC

Library of Congress Cataloging-in-Publication Data

Vigilante, Kevin.
    Low-fat lies, high-fat frauds, and the healthiest diet in the world / by Kevin Vigilante and Mary Flynn.
        p.   cm.
    Includes bibliographical references and index.
    ISBN 978-0-89526-220-2
     1. Nutrition. 2. Diet—Mediterranean Region. 3. Low-fat diet.
4. Low-carbohydrate diet.   I. Flynn, Mary. II. Title.
    RA784.V54 1999
    613.2—dc21   99–21204
                                             CIP

Published in the United States by
LifeLine Press
A Regnery Publishing Company
One Massachusetts Avenue, NW
Washington, DC 20001

Manufactured in the United States of America

Book design by Dori Miller
Medical Illustrations by Kevin Somerville

10

Books are available in quantity for promotional or premium use. Write to Director of Special Sales, Regnery Publishing, Inc., One Massachusetts Avenue, NW, Washington, DC 20001, for information on discounts and terms or call (202) 216-0600.

*We dedicate this book to the memory of
Giacomo Castelvetro, who first tried to save the English
from their food by introducing them to
the Mediterranean diet in 1614.*

Contents

Part Two: Good News from the Mediterranean

Part Three: Applying the Mediterranean Diet to Your Life

Acknowledgments

We would first like to thank our medical chiefs, Drs. Tim Flanigan and Charles Carpenter, for giving us the professional space to write a book for the popular press. We are also grateful to K. Dun Gifford of Oldways Preservation and Exchange Trust, not only for his support but for his vision. Francie King at Oldways helped us round up recipes from the members of Oldways's Chef's Collaborative; and thanks to the chefs who shared the secrets of their trade. Linda Russo and Diane Macher of the Olive Oil Council helped us track down arcane olive oil data, and Anne Kennedy Ilaqua from the Brown University Special Populations Library helped us track down even more arcane population, survival, and disease data. The following scholars we interviewed were most generous with their time and knowledge: Dr. Arthur Agatston from the Mount Sinai Medical Center in Miami, Dr. Ralph De Fronzo of the University of Texas–San Antonio, Dr. John Folts of the University of Wisconsin, Dr. John Freeman at Johns Hopkins Hospital, Dr. Mary Alice Kern from San Francisco State University, Dr. C. Lionis from the University of Crete, Dr. Steven McGarvey of Brown University, Dr. Carlos Muller at California State University at Fresno, Dr. Trudy Shephard from the University of Colorado, Dr. Dimitrios Trichopolous of the Harvard School of Public Health and the University of Athens, Dr. John Weisburger of the American Health Foundation, and finally Dr. Walter Willet of Harvard University, who was extraordinarily generous with his time and who has provided intellectually inspired leadership in the field of nutrition.

When it came to the nitty-gritty of getting the book edited and out the door, it's hard to say enough for the agile team at LifeLine Press. Erica Rogers, our chief editor, made this a much better book than the one we gave her. Trish Bozell, Jennifer Azar, Dori Miller, Marja Walker, and the imperturbable Dave Dortman all played an important part in the process. A special thanks to Richard Vigilante, who first encouraged us to write this book and who reworked several chapters.

We are extremely grateful to the employees of Brown University who came to our noontime lectures and helped us refine the weight-loss diet and recipes. Katherine Wright had the unenviable task of helping type the bibliography, and Christina Govatos helped with research.

Lastly and most importantly we want to thank our families for their support—especially our grandparents who came from distant shores and brought with them the peasants' wisdom of the old ways of eating.

Part One:
Low-Fat Lies and
High-Fat Frauds

1 A Matter of Life and Death

"**We** have a fifty-five-year-old man in full arrest, CPR in progress. We are three minutes out. Do you copy?" When the emergency medical technicians (EMTs) arrived we were waiting, fully gloved, in our appointed positions around the bed in the code bay. I was at the head of the bed, where I could take control of the airway and orchestrate the activity of the three nurses, two technicians, and the physician's assistant. Compressing the chest as the patient was rolled in, an EMT gave me the essentials: "Fifty-five-year-old male, no previous medical history, was at work and complained of feeling light-headed. He went down, and coworkers administered CPR. When we arrived he was in V-Fib so we shocked him. Got no pulse, so we shocked him again. Then he went flatline. Gave a total of seven milligrams of epinephrine but got nothing."

They counted to three, lifted together, and loaded his obese body on the emergency room gurney. I looked at his purple, plethoric face.

"How long before you guys got to him?" I asked.

"About ten minutes."

I passed a laryngoscope into his mouth, suctioned out the fluid and the vomit, and passed a tube into his trachea so we could deliver 100 percent oxygen directly to his lungs. I stood up from my stooped position. His large belly protruded each time they compressed his chest.

"And how long was his transport time?"

"About twenty minutes," the EMT responded.

Thirty minutes without a pulse. I knew then he wasn't going to make it. As soon as you go beyond eight to ten minutes, chances of survival plummet to near zero. But, you never know. So we continued to work on him. CPR, more epi (epinephrine), a flicker of chaotic heart activity, another shock, then flatline again.

His wife was already in the family room when I entered. She knew what I was going to say, but still she looked at me with fearful, expectant eyes that said, "Don't tell me that. I don't want to hear that. Tell me something different."

I sat down, and as I took her hand she knew the inevitable was coming and started to cry.

"I'm very sorry."

The sobs grew louder.

"He passed on."

She wailed. "No, no, he didn't. Don't tell me that. It's not true."

"I'm sorry, ma'am. We did everything we could."

"What happened?"

"It looks like he had a massive heart attack," I said. "He went very quickly, even before the rescue squad got there. I can assure you that he didn't suffer."

"But he was fine," she said. "He had no problems. He just saw the doctor two months ago. He was going to retire and we were going to...." She couldn't finish the sentence.

"I know, I know," I said, although I knew he couldn't have been fine. This problem had been brewing silently for years.

"I guess it was his time," she said.

"I guess it was." But I didn't really believe that. It's a great comfort to the grieving to believe the hour of death is beyond our control. I suppose sometimes it is. But after seeing too many premature deaths from gunshot wounds, drug abuse, drunk driving, smoking, overeating, and sedentary living, I long ago stopped believing that we are passive victims of fate. Many people who end up in the emergency room make choices that land them there.

The patient's wife composed herself, picked up the phone, and dialed. But when she made the connection she barely got the words out. "Daddy's gone. He's dead." She started crying again. Saying the words to someone else always seems to make it more real, more final. "I'm with the doctor now. Yes, yes, I'm fine." Then she hung up, put her head down, and sobbed the deep, quiet cry of someone who had lost her best friend and was facing the rest of her life alone.

You remember some resuscitations better than others. I don't know why this one from years ago sticks in my mind, but it does. Maybe it's because his wife was so sweet. I must confess that I don't remember their names. I do know that I have had such conversations too many times in nearly twenty years in medicine.

Most of the premature deaths I see are preventable. This man was fifty to seventy-five pounds overweight. He could have dramatically lowered his risk by making relatively simple changes in his lifestyle. Instead, because of his central obesity (obesity concentrated around the midsection), he had been set up for what is called the *metabolic syndrome*. This syndrome, which is epidemic in our society, consists of obesity, abnormal levels of cholesterol and triglycerides (blood fats), high blood pressure, elevated fasting insulin, and a predisposition to blood clotting. Often these abnormalities are subtle and, taken individually, might be overlooked. But combined they can do tremendous damage over the years and eventually choke off the blood vessels feeding the heart.

What could he have done to put off that day and enjoy another twenty or thirty years with his family? You know the answer. Diet and exercise. Now you'll turn off, tune out, and give up, because you've heard it too many times before and tried too many times before, and you are tired of failing.

But don't give up yet. Yes, diet and exercise are the key. That much of what you've heard is true. But if you are the typical American listening to the typical advice that you get from doctors, dietitians, the media, and food manufacturers, you have been set up for failure. In fact, you've been lied to. Maybe not on purpose, and sometimes with good intentions, but the bottom line is that you haven't been told the truth. And the truth is that the diet regimen embraced by most physicians, the National Cholesterol Education Program, and low-fat gurus such as Dr. Dean Ornish largely haven't worked for most people.

If you are one of tens of millions of Americans who have tried and failed to lower your weight, maintain an exercise program, or control your cholesterol, the reason may be that you have been programmed to fail. In all likelihood the dietary advice you have been given is fundamentally flawed, is impractical for most people, requires radical and unpalatable changes, and is simply impossible for most people to stick with.

If you are like the majority of Americans who have been programmed to fail in this way, you have been the victim of *low-fat lies.*

For most of you the core of your dietary program is a radical reduction in fat intake. For almost thirty years Americans have been cutting back on fat, or trying to. The percentage of fat in the American diet has dropped by almost 15 percent, and low-fat prepared foods litter the grocery shelves. And all this time Americans have continued to get fatter—over 30 percent fatter.

If that's your story, you've been victimized by the *low-fat lie.* Tens of millions probably have been victimized in this way over the past thirty years. The truth is, not only do low-fat diets often not work, for many people who fail to lose weight they may actually be dangerous, worsening HDL cholesterol and triglycerides. Very low-fat diets may even deprive the body of important nutrients that defend against heart disease and cancer.

The low-fat diet craze has been with us for two decades, yet Americans continue to gain weight. Why? The reason is simple: Much of the time, low-fat diets don't work.

Low-fat diets are unsatisfying, unpalatable, and for most people impossible to stick to. And there is compelling new evidence that they can be positively unhealthy.

If a low-fat diet is good, a very-low-fat diet must be better, and a no-fat diet must be best of all, right? After years of low-fat propaganda, many seem to think so. The no-fat/low-fat message has become so pervasive that in a poll of schoolchildren, 81 percent thought that the healthiest diet possible is one that eliminated all dietary fat—a nutritional disaster.

Americans have been convinced that "low fat" is synonymous with "healthy." They treat fat like poison, and they are obsessed with banishing it from their lives. They will eat a cupboard full of rice cakes for lunch and pasta by the pound for dinner and wonder why they don't lose weight. Even if they do lose weight on the very-low-fat diets recommended by low-fat gurus, they have a hard time sticking to the diet and keeping off the weight. Worse yet, and unknown to them, if they fail to lose weight, as many do, their low-fat diets may be causing dangerous biochemical side effects that may increase the health risks low-fat diets are intended to reduce—a danger they will seldom hear about from Nathan Pritikin, Dr. Dean Ornish, and other fat phobes.

> Not only do low-fat diets not work, they may actually be dangerous, worsening HDL cholesterol and triglycerides.

These days there is a new lie out there, just as dangerous as the old one, that a lot of people are falling for because of their frustration with the failure of low-fat diets.

Maybe you are one of them. Maybe in frustration you have turned to the super-high-fat Atkins diet or its cousins, the Zone and Sugar Busters diets. But these unproven fad diets are just as flawed as the low-fat advice that drove you to try them. In fact, the Atkins diet is potentially so dangerous that the surgeon general should probably put a warning on every book Dr. Robert Atkins sells. The diet's only salvation is that people can't tolerate it for very long—not long enough for the increase in the risk of heart disease or cancer that long-term use of such a diet could bring.

Low-fat lies. High-fat frauds. Both are perpetuated by misinformation propagated by government, doctors, the media, and various health organizations. Are they out to get you? Do they mean you harm? No, but most of the nutritional advice Americans get is distorted by one disastrous assumption made by well-intentioned experts: Most people are not smart enough to really understand everything they need to know to take control of their own nutrition and health. So the experts feed us half-truths like "avoid fat," because they think we can't understand the real, somewhat more complex message.

And all the time Americans keep getting fatter. The production of diet foods, books, and advice—almost all based on gross over-simplifications—has become an industry bigger than the gross domestic product of a small country. And so Americans continue to gain weight, eat badly, and suffer from the chronic diseases associated with obesity and poor nutrition.

The most egregious violations of truth can be found in the legions of diet books that peddle distorted information to an unsuspecting and vulnerable public. These modern-day snake-oil salesmen should be condemned to the first circle of dieters' inferno. Right next to them are the food manufacturers that exploit our cultural obsession with fat to convince folks that their highly unhealthy, calorie-dense, processed foods are good for you because they are low in fat. In the next circle go those who present shaky theory as fact. There is nothing wrong with having hunches and opinions, but if that's what they are, they should be identified as such. In matters of health it is irresponsible to present unproven theory as fact, no matter how good it sounds on paper. That's how people get hurt. In dieters' purgatory go the well-intentioned medical professionals and health agencies who want very much to do the right thing but who, for a variety of reasons, have fallen victim to lies, myths, or misinformation.

So, is there no hope? Actually, there is hope. You can dramatically improve your prospects. You can lose weight; improve your blood pressure and blood lipids; lower your risk of stroke, heart disease, and cancer; and increase your chances of living a long, healthy life without ever eating another rice cake, going on a dangerous fad diet, eating cottage cheese with lettuce every day, or becoming a lifelong gym rat.

For the most part you can do it without "dieting" in the conventional American sense. This book will show you how. "Knowledge is power," a wise man once said, and we are going to give you the power to use food in a healthy, happy way. By the time you're finished, you will know enough so that you will no longer be trapped by mindless rituals of fad diets that make you a slave to food—or some diet doctor's bizarre, unappetizing notion of what food is. You will learn how to love and respect food, eat healthier, enjoy food more than you ever have before, and take control of food and make it the core of your own way of healthy living. You will learn about one of the healthiest diets in the world—not a diet in the conventional sense but a way of life (which is what the word "diet" originally meant).

This diet has worked for thousands of years, producing some of the lowest rates of cancer, heart disease, stroke, and other chronic diseases of aging in the world. But only in recent years has a number of scientists unearthed the true reasons for the power unleashed by adopting this way of life. What these scientists have learned is very different from most of the dietary advice most Americans have been getting for many years.

Obesity is epidemic in America and around the world. Even in far-off places more often associated with privation and hunger, obesity is spreading along with the proliferation of modern technology and lifestyles. It is a life-threatening epidemic spreading the diseases of modern life—cancer, diabetes, kidney failure, hypertension, heart disease, arthritis, and others. By the time patients arrive in the emergency room blue and without a pulse, it is too late. The time to prevent these needless premature deaths is now. And the best way to do that is to stop smoking, eat right, exercise, and lose weight.

But you can't eat right or lose weight if you hate food. Food is a central pleasure in life. No dogmatic directive from any doctor or diet guru is going to change that by telling you everything will be okay if you just switch to the latest bizarre, unpalatable diet.

Let's face it: A life of fat-free muffins, fat-free salad dressing, fat-free chocolate chip "un"cookies, tofu, and raw broccoli is, well, not worth living. The proof: Nobody lives that way. Our diets don't last because we hate them. They are not a permanent part of a good life but rather our temporary penance for "too much of a good thing." Any prescription for attacking the epidemic of obesity has to respect our universal human propensity to celebrate and enjoy food. People will not adhere to diets that require a lifetime of privation. There are certain cultures that are particularly renowned for their love affair with food and have very low rates of heart disease, cancer, stroke, and the other diseases of modern life. The Mediterranean cultures, in particular, celebrate food with intense passion—and they have some of the lowest rates of these diseases in the world. The truth is, the more we know food, love food, and respect food, and all the celebrations and rituals that go with food, the thinner and healthier we will be.

Dr. Dean Ornish and Dr. Robert Atkins can't help you, because no matter what they say, they hate food. Ornish practically bans half of all the possible foods you could eat (foods with fat), and Atkins bans the other half (foods with carbohydrates).

We truly love food. True love implies not just passion and affection but respect and reverence as well. Rekindling reverence for food isn't hard, and it isn't time consuming, but it does require awareness, thought, and some reflection. In this book we will present a good deal of scientific information about diet, weight loss, health, and nutrition. We also provide practical guidelines to help you achieve your health and weight-loss goals, including some quick, simple recipes for healthy and delicious eating. But we hope that we also impart a sense of reverence for the food that, in a very real and miraculous way, becomes you. Such reverence for food is vitally important to achieving health and weight loss.

Although we have passion and reverence for food, we do not have similar feelings about protein, carbohydrates, or fat. These are not foods. As food reformer Dun Gifford is fond of pointing out, "You don't say, 'Honey, let's go out tonight and have some carbohydrates.' When you go to the store, you don't walk down the fat aisle or protein aisle."

But that's what the diet gurus want you to do. That's even what the National Cancer Institute and the National Cholesterol Education Program want you to do. And that's one reason why their advice fails.

When we talk about what we want to eat, we talk about real foods: grilled trout, pasta puttanesca, arugula salad, risotto with sun-dried tomatoes, tomatoes with mozzarella and olive oil, mussels in white wine sauce, spinach and bean soup, baked potatoes, grilled vegetables, a smooth merlot, a succulent peach. These are foods. They feed our bodies and souls. They are shared with family and friends. They mark the great moments in our lives—birthdays, graduations, and weddings. But they are also part of our daily routine. By passionately and reverently making the right foods part of our daily routine, we will be much healthier and happier. Any strategy for a lifetime of health and weight control must be based on the simple recognition that people by their nature are drawn to food.

Unfortunately our national strategy for health and weight control is not based on food but on nutrients. Actually, today, it is based on only one nutrient—fat. Aristotle said, "Small mistakes in the beginning can lead to enormous errors in the end." This has certainly proven to be the case in America. The narrow-minded focus on fat has been a failure that seems to have exacerbated the problem of obesity. The people who have profited are food manufacturers and certain diet-book authors who have exploited the well-intended but poorly conceived government guidelines. They have used the no-fat/low-fat label as a governmental imprimatur meant to be synonymous with health and weight loss.

This corruption of the government's seemingly simple message to consume less than 30 percent of your diet as fat has spawned decades of lies, myths, and misconceptions about what and how much people should eat. And now, with the obvious failure of the narrow focus on fat, there has been a recent pendulum swing among popular diet books. The new best-selling message is that the problem isn't fat at all but sugar and other carbohydrates. Although the success of this latest round of books seems to be in direct proportion to the failure of the low-fat strategy, this new message is equally flawed because, once again, it fails to focus on real food and relies instead on bizarre, unpalatable diets no one will stick to.

To make matters worse, the government can't even get its story straight. While government health agencies keep mouthing the low-fat mantra, the U.S. Department of Agriculture pushes meat consumption through its famous food pyramid created under the careful watch of the powerful cattle and beef lobby.

I don't know the personal habits of the unfortunate man who

died in the emergency room that day. But I do know that he was obese and that his obesity put him at high risk for disease and death. If he was like most Americans, his doctor probably told him to lose weight and go on a low-fat diet. But despite the low-fat ice cream, yogurt, chips, cheese, salad dressing, pretzels, and cookies, he just got fatter and fatter. As he did, his levels of good cholesterol fell, his triglyceride levels climbed, and his fasting insulin levels rose. Without exercise and adequate doses of antioxidants provided by fruits and vegetables, the process progressed unchecked. As it did the deposits inside his blood vessels got thicker and thicker until they choked off the blood supply to his heart. That's when he collapsed, his heart stopped beating, he turned purple, and he died. Even though his wife indulged herself in the self-deception that it was his preordained time, and even though I was a silent accomplice to her deception, this tragically premature death could have been prevented. Although it is too late for him, it is not too late for you and millions of other Americans. It is for you and for them that this book is written.

Americans are constantly confronted with lies, misconceptions, and myths about diet. Today, confusion reigns because juxtaposed to the low-fat fanatics is an equally fanatic faction urging dieters to eat as much fat—any fat—as they can get their hands on. No wonder Americans are confused. In the course of this book, we go beyond the lie of the low-fat diet to expose high-fat frauds, clear up carbohydrate conundrums, and present you with a time-tested way to achieve health by eating truly delicious and satisfying food. We will show you the following:

■   Why low-fat diets so often fail when it comes to permanent weight loss.

■ How the latest in medical research—including research by coauthor Dr. Mary Flynn—exposes the false promises and potential risks of low-fat diets.

■ How low-fat diets can worsen the levels of dangerous blood fats you never hear about (triglycerides).

■ How the diet recommended by the National Cholesterol Education Program can worsen your cholesterol and triglyceride levels if you fail to lose weight.

■ How extremely low-fat diets might deprive you of valuable nutrients that may help prevent heart disease, stroke, and cancer.

■ How pizza may help prevent prostate cancer.

■ What nutritional benefits the foods that make up the Mediterranean diet provide.

■ How to tell good fats from bad fats, and how the right kinds of fat are essential to good nutrition and health, and can help reduce levels of bad cholesterol (LDL) and dangerous triglycerides.

■ How eating the right kind of fat may help lower your risk of breast cancer.

■ Why a popular no-fat diet food may be one of the most unhealthy items in your fridge. (Hint: It comes in a bottle and you shake before pouring.)

■ How olive oil can raise levels of good cholesterol without increasing bad cholesterol; can reduce dangerous triglyceride levels; and may help to lower the risk of cancer.

■ How another fat—this one from the sea—can prevent

the arterial blockages and blood clots that cause strokes and heart disease.

■ How in one of the healthiest nations on earth the average person's diet is almost 40 percent fat—but the right kind of fat.

■ What your doctor probably doesn't know about the true effects—and dangers—of low-fat diets, blood lipids, and the low-fat craze.

■ What fats really are risky—including those the government, under the influence of food lobbies, are encouraging Americans to consume.

■ Why the government's food pyramid, which you see displayed on the walls of doctors' offices, in schools, and even on cereal boxes, is hazardous to your health.

■ How the most potentially deadly fat of all is being pushed into your diet—especially your children's—and how to get it out of your home and your life.

■ Why the very high-fat fad diets may often be dangerous.

■ How to get the exercise you need without becoming a gym rat.

■ How you can embrace one of the healthiest diets in the world, eat better than ever before, start a love affair with food—and still lose weight.

■ How you can fuse the wisdom of ancient cultures with modern science to embrace a diet and way of life that will help you reach your potential for health and longevity.

Much of what we say will be controversial because we criticize many of the mandarins of medicine and nutrition. It's not that they are *all* wrong, and they certainly are not liars in the literal sense, but many have become personally or institutionally invested in certain points of view that are proving with new research to be erroneous. Rather than admit error or entertain alternatives, they often go through intellectual contortions to defend those positions.

We propose a different approach. We will endeavor to provide information that addresses the nuances and subtleties of food, nutrition, fat, and obesity. At times learning this information requires some science and some effort. But we think that your time and effort will be well spent, and we are confident that people will invest the effort because they are hungry for the truth. But we also recognize that food is not reducible to chemical equations. Food is about nourishment on many levels, both physical and psychological. It is about pleasure, art, taste, and aesthetics. It is about family, friends, and love. Though Mary Flynn has a Ph.D. in nutrition and I am a physician, we are food lovers in the fullest sense of the term. Not only has Flynn made a career out of studying food, she also grows it, cooks it, celebrates it, and thoroughly enjoys eating it. I love food so much my brother and I opened our own restaurant, Christopher Martins, in New Haven, Connecticut. Our objective is to provide food lovers with the scientific tools to better understand the foods they love and to prove to them that they don't have to surrender these foods to be healthy.

Low-Fat Lies not only exposes the diet myths and clears up the confusion, it also offers an alternative: a delicious, satisfying, and healthy way of eating and *living*. It shows you how to use the right fats well, adjust your diet in other pleasant and positive ways, and alter your thinking and lifestyle in ways that will reduce stress and increase fitness without arduous and impractical exercise regimens. You can be healthy, lose weight, and enjoy food—and life—again.

2 Why Low-Fat Diets Don't Work

Y ou've been on a low-fat diet once, twice, maybe even three times, and now, as you read these words, you are just as overweight as when you started. Frustrating, isn't it? Especially when you are bombarded with information about the need to eat less fat to lose weight. You can't walk down the aisle of a food store without being assaulted with thousands of labels that proclaim "Low Fat!" or "No Fat!" Into the cart they go. You eat them, and you often gain more weight.

Have you ever wondered, "If everyone else can lose weight by cutting fat, what's wrong with me?" Well, the fact is that there is nothing wrong with you. Millions of Americans have been eating less fat and getting fatter. The problem isn't you; the problem is the sound-bite, made-for-TV message: "Eat less fat and you will be less fat."

Don't be embarrassed that you got sucked in. The low-fat propaganda has most of us believing that fat calories in food lead directly to fat on our bodies. It's like Rhoda's line on the old *Mary Tyler Moore Show*: "I don't know why I am eating this; I should just apply it directly to my hips."

But not only do most Americans believe it, most of the country's doctors, dietitians, and health organizations do too. For years our most respected health organizations pumped out that message. The American Heart Association diet guidelines have called "restriction of fat intake... the cornerstone of these dietary recommendations." For years the government's National Cholesterol Education Program has been popularizing the idea that eating less fat leads to weight loss and recommends diets in which fat is less than 30 percent of total calories.

But low-fat diets as commonly conceived do not work, can be medically harmful, and do not represent the best diet for many people—especially if they want to lose weight and keep it off.

Discovering the Lie

Physicians in general know precious little about the fine points of nutrition. We learn about biochemistry and metabolic function but get very little training in how to apply that knowledge to the foods people actually eat. There is no medical specialty in nutrition, and outside our area of expertise, we physicians are just as likely as most Americans to be victims of information overload and communication by sound bite.

So, like most Americans, I was a low-fat fanatic for years (without being especially thin!). I was convinced from what I had read that no diet was too low in fat. I preached it to my overweight patients, and I tried to practice it myself. But I had a hard time sticking to the program. Either I hated the food or I was hungry all the time. My patients, friends, and family had similar problems. Nevertheless, I kept exhorting them to get with the program, and I kept reading labels, calculating fat grams, and eating rice cakes.

Then I returned to Italy, where I had lived years before, for a vacation. I went, I saw, I ate. I showed no restraint. I saw no food labeled "no fat," and almost everything I ate was awash in olive oil. I walked quite a bit, but I wasn't exercising any more than usual. To my surprise, when I got home I felt my clothes were looser. Then I got on the scale. I had lost almost five pounds.

> Low-fat diets do not work, can be medically harmful, and do not represent the best diet for many people—especially if they want to lose weight and keep it off.

I casually mentioned my "miraculous" weight loss to my nutritionist colleague, Dr. Mary Flynn. She wasn't surprised at all. "Sure, a little fat helps you lose weight."

I was shocked. It seemed too good to be true. My Irish half just couldn't accept the notion that you could lose weight without immense suffering.

She said, "I don't believe in low-fat diets. They just don't work. Fat makes food taste good, and it makes you feel full. Without a little fat you're always going to be hungry."

I thought about all those cheddar-flavored rice cakes in my cupboard and nodded with the knowledge of one who had known hunger.

"The key," she said, "is to eat the right kind of fat, in the right amounts. You have to build it into your diet, like the Greeks and Italians do." Flynn read my doubt. "You can always lose weight temporarily," she said. "The question is how to keep it off for a lifetime. That's where these fad diets and low-fat diets typically fail. You need a diet you can live with. You need some fat in your diet."

That was my first introduction to the low-fat lie.

As we talked, I learned that Flynn had done her Ph.D. dissertation on the frequent failure of low-fat diets and their health risks. With her encouragement I made a study of nutrition and diets, using Flynn's extensive files. The picture became clear: The right fats in the right quantity are crucial to optimizing health and shedding excess pounds.

The Taste Test

Taste is vital to the success of any diet. Ironically, this is a big reason fat phobes fear fat so much. Fat tastes good. Fat phobes are afraid people will overconsume it and put on weight, so their alternative is low-fat diets. In effect, they are saying, "If we give people low-fat diets they won't like the taste and won't overeat." Interesting strategy. But common sense tells you that most people aren't going to stay on that diet very long. And even though some people temporarily lose weight on low-fat diets, before too long they often find themselves indulging in a fat-feeding frenzy— often with the kind of fats that are most unhealthy. Sometimes dieters substitute large quantities of sugar for the low-fat taste deficit. Either way, the low-fat diet then fails and they end up putting on more weight.

Fat phobes base this "passive overconsumption" argument on experiments with mice and humans that have shown when fat is slipped into food, more calories are consumed. But there are some problems with these experiments: First, humans consciously choose what to eat, and eating behavior is often modified when information about food is available. Knowing the calorie or fat content of food is important to how much food people consume. For instance, if you tell a group that a certain yogurt is low fat and one is high fat, they will tend to eat *more* of what they think is low fat. Other experiments show that people who think they are eating a low-calorie meal will often eat more at their next meal.

This has a couple of implications. One is that mouse-feeding experiments may hold little meaning for humans—mice don't think much about food. The other is that there may be a big difference between hidden fat (fat you can't see like in a donut) as opposed to visible (fat you can see and measure like oil). The world's healthiest high-fat diets use visible fats like olive oil that are consciously added to foods and can be precisely measured. With visible fats it is obvious how much fat you are using. That knowledge can modify how much you consume. Some of the world's unhealthiest diets are dominated by hidden fats. In America the biggest source of fat is hidden fat in ground meat. Pastries are another big source of hidden fat. It is much easier to overconsume hidden fats, usually in the form of saturated fats—the unhealthiest kind. Most fat research fails to account for this.

Another issue fat phobes frequently bring up is that fat is energy dense, that is, it has more calories per ounce than carbohydrates or protein (twice as many to be precise). But that's what *makes* it palatable. Research shows that foods with high energy density like chocolate, peanut butter, french fries, or olive oil simply taste better to most people than foods that have low energy density like spinach, broccoli, asparagus, or rice.

But this is no reason to ban foods that taste good. It makes more sense to harness that palatability to make other healthy foods—for instance, spinach is more delicious by adding a little olive oil. This is what enables the healthiest Mediterranean countries to consume such vast quantities of low-calorie, disease fighting vegetables—the palatability imparted to them by healthy, visible fats.

The bottom line is that people won't eat food they don't like for very long, but adding some healthy fat to your diet, like olive oil can make boring, low-calorie vegetables absolutely delicious.

Feeling Full

Not only do low-fat diets not taste good, they often leave us hungry. Achieving satiety or feeling full involves a number of complex biological and psychological factors and is not completely understood, but we know that fats, fiber, carbohydrates, and protein all play a role. Leave any one of them out of your diet (most fad diets ignore at least one) and you are likely to feel hungry sooner than you would normally.

The key is to eat the right kind of fat, in the right amounts— build it into your diet, like the Greeks and Italians do.

For instance, carbohydrates, especially fiber, literally fill you up. The physical distention of the stomach produced by these bulky foods, like spinach and broccoli, sends a signal to the brain telling you to stop eating. But the effects of distention don't last long, and even if you were able to eat enough unadorned broccoli to temporarily distend your stomach before unbearable monotony set in, without a little fat you'd be hungry again in no time. That's when you reach for the Ben and Jerry's before going to bed.

The effects of fat on feeling full tend to show up after a few hours rather than soon after eating. In one study a group of volunteers were given high-fat and low-fat breakfasts. Those who ate the high-fat breakfast felt full longer and postponed the time of the next meal (this may be important in helping you avoid those calorie packed mid-afternoon or late-night snacks). Eating fat stimulates the release of a hormone that slows the rate of food leaving the stomach, causing you to feel full longer. The small intestine also has fat receptors that, when stimulated by fat, send signals to the brain making you feel full.

Palatability (good taste) and satiety (feeling full) are actually opposing forces. Highly palatable foods, like chocolate ice cream, taste so good that we may continue eating even though we feel full. Other less tasty foods, like bland rice or raw broccoli, may fill us up temporarily and are less tempting to overeat; but who can bear a lifetime of eating such boring, unpalatable foods?

The solution for healthy living and weight loss is not penitential low-fat diets devoid of taste. The answer is to use healthy fats wisely so food tastes good *and* fills you up. The truth is that when used properly, fat can be an important ally to help you lose weight and keep it off. And that's what the Mediterranean diet does so well.

The Frustration Factor

Another reason low-fat diets fail is sheer frustration. The government says you're supposed to consume less than 30 percent of your calories from fat. But any diet that requires such complicated calculations is destined to fail. It's one thing to count calories, but low-fat diets require you to divide, multiply, and figure out percentages of fat calories.

We asked physicians to tell us how many grams of fat a 150-pound man consuming a 2,000-calorie, 30-percent-fat diet should eat. More than a third got the answer wrong. If doctors can't figure out the correct answer, how are you supposed to calculate it when you're sitting in a restaurant?

Scientific Evidence

So why is the scientific establishment so gaga over low-fat diets? You would think there must be overwhelming proof that such diets are the key to weight loss, health, and longevity. The truth is just the opposite: *There is no conclusive proof that eating higher-fat diets causes obesity.*

Dueling Fat Facts

Fat phobes like Dr. Dean Ornish often cite research showing that it takes more energy to store carbohydrates in fat cells than it does to store dietary fat in fat cells. They conclude that if you eat 200 calories from butter and 200 from bread, the 200 from butter will make you fatter. But it's *calories* that count, not where they come from that matters. Basing elaborate theories on single biochemical pathways leads to error because there are thousands of biochemical reactions going on in the body at any given moment.

Ornish and others fail to point out that:

- Researchers from Canada found that animals fed low-fat diets produce increased amounts of a fat-making enzyme.

- Researchers from the Rockefeller University found that people on very-low-fat diets manufacture fat at a dramatically increased rate. So eating less fat actually can cause your body to make more.

- Researchers from the University of Colorado found that when people go on low-fat diets, a fat storage enzyme called lipoprotein lipase becomes more active, causing the small amount of fat you are eating to be stored more easily, thereby potentially increasing fat storage in the body.

Does this nullify the efficiency argument that Ornish embraces? Maybe, but maybe not. The point is you can't seize upon a single biochemical observation to prove how the body will react to a particular nutrient. This is a common problem in fad diets like the Atkins, Zone, and Sugar Busters diets. The scientific evidence indicates that caloric intake is the key to weight gain. Whether these calories come from tofu or chocolate toffee is irrelevant.

Population Studies

What about direct scientific evidence from real people? There are basically two types of experimental evidence, and neither proves the low-fat position.

The first type is derived from a comparison of whole populations. Such a comparison is called an epidemiological study.

For instance, fat phobes point out that in China, people eat very little fat and the Chinese, on average, are less obese than Europeans. But such a comparison proves nothing. Europe is much richer than China. Food of all sorts—fat and carbohydrate—is more abundant in Europe, and Europeans eat more and get less exercise than the Chinese. Sitting around and eating too much, not the percentage of fat in their diets, are the likely reasons why Europeans (and Americans) are chubbier.

It would be more valid to compare individuals in similar cultures. A researcher named Lauren Lissner did just that when she examined fat consumption and obesity among Europeans. She found that in diets ranging from about 25 percent to 47 percent fat there was no relationship between the percentage of fat consumed and the level of obesity in men. As for women, there was actually an inverse relationship: The higher the percentage of fat in the diet, the less likely the women were to be obese! Drs. Chen Junshi and Colin Campbell took a similar approach when they studied obesity rates in 65 different counties in China. Even though fat intake in the counties ranged from 8 percent to 25 percent, they could find no correlation between fat intake and body weight.

On the whole, the evidence shows little proof that eating fat makes you fatter than eating the same amount of calories in carbohydrates or proteins.

Randomized Human Diet Experiments

The other source of experimental evidence from real people is from so-called randomized human experiments, which simply means that researchers put two randomly chosen groups of people on two different diets, watch them very closely, and then compare the results. Once again, such studies do not prove the anti-fat position. What they do show is that the anti-fat position is not nearly as strong as the rhetoric suggests and there is ample reason to pursue other strategies. They also show that proponents of low-fat diets should temper their enthusiasm with the doubt that is suggested by the evidence. That would be the more honest thing to do.

These studies can be divided into short-term studies, one week to six months, and long-term studies, six months to years. Some, but not all, short-term studies do show that people on low-fat diets tend to lose more weight, though the difference is quite modest. For instance, in another study by Dr. Lissner, people were allowed to eat freely from a high-fat menu or a low-fat menu in a research kitchen. At the end of this fourteen-day study those consuming the low-fat foods lost slightly more weight. However, neither this study nor any of the studies like it examines whether hidden fat calories are more likely to be accidently overconsumed than visible fat calories like those from olive oil, which can easily be seen or measured. Finally, people who lost weight on this study consumed fewer calories, and so it doesn't support the notion that fat calories are, in themselves, more fattening than carboyhdrate calories.

Coauthor Mary Flynn did an experiment in which she placed subjects on low-fat and high-fat diets with identical calorie counts. She found that weights were no different in either group, high-fat or low-fat.

> Fat can be an important ally to help you lose weight and keep it off.

The weights changed only when she randomly assigned subjects to diets with different total calories. She found what many others have found in short randomized studies: It's total calories that count, not whether they come from fat or carbohydrates.

The more crucial question is not what happens in the short term—lots of us can lose weight temporarily—but what happens in the long term. There are only a handful of long-term studies examining low-fat diets and weight loss because they are quite expensive and difficult to do. But among the handful that do exist they generally show that in the first few months people tend to lose a few more pounds on a low-fat diet, but then, perhaps when overcome by the boredom of a low-palatability diet, they tend to put the weight back on. At the end of a year or two the differences between the lower- and higher-fat diets are generally negligible. To cast even more doubt on the anemic effect of these low-fat diets, in almost all cases those receiving them got more coaching and counseling. In the National Heart Diet Study, one of the most rigorous long-term studies, both the high- and low-fat groups were treated identically with regard to coaching and counseling, and at the end of a year the low-fat group only had a two-pound advantage. Hardly a slam-dunk for low-fat diets, and not the kind of evidence you want to build national policy on. Yet, we have.

The frequent failure of very-low-fat diets is well illustrated in a recent study published in the *Journal of the American Medical Association* in 1998. In this year-long study, four groups of highly motivated men were randomly assigned to one of four diets containing 18, 22, 26, or 30 percent fat with the same number of calories. This study demonstrated a number of things. First, the men on the 18- and 22-percent-fat diets had a hard time sticking to the plan. They ended up consuming 22- and 24-percent-fat diets, respectively. (Even highly motivated dieters, under close supervision, have trouble sticking to low-fat diets.)

The study also showed that those consuming 22 percent fat lost no more weight than those consuming 30 percent fat—showing again that it's calories that count the most, not whether those calories come from fat or carbohydrates.

In 1998 Walter Willet, chairman of the department of nutrition at the Harvard School of Public Health, surveyed the scientific literature on dietary fat and obesity in far more detail than we can here, but his conclusion was similar to ours: "Diets high in fat do not appear to be the primary cause of the high prevalence of excess body fat in our society, and reductions in fat will not be a solution."

Death by Snackwells

In the late 1970s, just about the time the low-fat craze was getting started, Americans got an average of 40 percent of their calories from fat. By the mid-1990s that figure was down to 34 percent. Yet over the same time the percentage of obese Americans soared by more than 30 percent. This is particularly striking when you consider that in the previous twenty years obesity had increased by less than 5 percent. After the medical definition of obesity was

Comparison of Foods with Low-Fat Versions

	CALORIES	FAT GRAMS
Oreos (3 cookies)	160	7
Reduced-Fat Oreos (3 cookies)	130	3.5
Cracker Jacks (28g)	120	2
Fat-Free Cracker Jacks (28g)	110	0
Nilla Wafers (8 wafers)	140	5
Reduced-Fat Nilla Wafers (8 wafers)	120	2
Wheat Thins (29g)	140	6
Reduced-Fat Wheat Thins (29g)	120	4
Triscuits (31g/7 Triscuits)	140	5
Reduced-Fat Triscuits (32g/8 Triscuits)	130	3
Jif, Creamy (2 tbsp.)	190	16
Reduced-Fat Jif, Creamy (2 tbsp.)	190	12

changed in 1998, approximately 50 percent of all Americans were suddenly considered obese. But how can Americans be getting fatter on low-fat diets? Quite simply, we are pigging out on low-fat foods under the false assumption that "low fat" equals weight loss and health while "high fat" equals weight gain and disease. But that's not true, and low-fat products have almost as many calories as the regular-fat versions.

Double Deception

These foods are doubly deceptive and doubly damaging. Research has shown that when folks know something is "low fat," they are likely to either eat more of it or eat it in order to justify a Boston cream pie.

In 1990 the U.S. government challenged food manufacturers to come up with five thousand low-fat food products by the year 2000. They came up with almost six thousand by 1993. We're not talking about asparagus spears here; we're talking about low-fat Chips Ahoy cookies. The National Cholesterol Education Program is still encouraging these commercial low-fat or "fat-modified" products, and the American Heart Association says these highly processed, low-fat products can make low-fat diets "much easier and more fun." Well they may be "more fun," but coupled with a sedentary lifestyle, these calorie-packed, low-fat products may be killing us.

Since the 1970s, Americans have added an extra 28 pounds of sugar a year to their diets. These extra sugar calories add up to approximately 49,000 extra calories per person, which, barring added exercise, means an extra 14 pounds of body fat. That's not the teaspoon of sugar you put in your coffee. It's the tons of sugar you don't even know about that are buried in commercial low-fat foods. And that's just the sugar. It doesn't include the tons of extra carbohydrates people feel free to consume because they are eating "fat-free foods." The kicker, of course, is that Americans are even more sedentary than in the 1970s. Nielsen ratings reveal that Americans spend over 15 percent more time in front of the TV. They also spend countless more hours playing video games and surfing the Internet. Commercial low-fat foods and TV go together like obesity and a heart attack.

Summing Up Fat Phobia

Despite the limited scientific evidence supporting the long-term efficacy of low-fat diets and despite their obvious failure in the real world, fat phobia remains rampant. With the exception of the American Diabetes Association, most official health agencies remain monolithically and dogmatically anti-fat. First-rate scientific and health organizations like the American Heart Association, the government's National Cholesterol Education Program, the National Cancer Institute, and the American Dietetic Association, as well as the vast majority of physicians, all seem to be telling us to stay away from fat because it will make us fat. Their admonitions often come in bold, sweeping, oversimplified statements that would lead one to assume that the evidence that fat causes obesity is as strong as the evidence that smoking causes cancer. Hardly. Nevertheless, the absolute dominance of this distorted message has convinced 81 percent of schoolchildren that the healthiest diet is one with no fat in it at all. Nothing could be further from the truth—and American schoolchildren, by the way, have never been fatter.

3 Diets That Do Work

I t has been said that no diets—high-fat or low-fat—work. Well, that's only half true. As Bill Clinton might say, it depends on what you mean by "diet."

Diet comes from the Greek word for routine, *diaita*, and from the Latin word for habit, *diaeta*. So diet is either

1) a regimen imposed for a specific purpose—like weight loss, or

2) a daily habit or way of living.

Diets under the first definition almost always fail. The National Institute of Health technology assessment conference panel estimated their failure rate at almost 100 percent after five years. Many of these failed diets are low-fat diets.

The second definition of diet is radically different. It describes a way of eating that develops organically, usually over centuries of cultural and culinary evolution. It is neither temporary nor extreme and carries with it the wisdom of age. We speak of Asian diets, Dutch diets, Greek diets, Italian diets, and English diets. But it would be even more accurate to describe diets according to a region such as Provence in France or Calabria in Italy. These diets are a union of the natural and cultural ecology of the region. Not all of these diets are equally healthy, but each is a way of eating that is seamlessly and organically intertwined with life. Today, according to anthropologist Sidney Mintz of Johns Hopkins University, there is no "American diet," national or regional, in this sense of the word.

> You can enjoy good food, *and* lose weight, *and* improve your health.

We don't question whether culturally evolved diets are successful or unsuccessful, or whether people can "stick" to them. People don't try to "stick to" their regional diets because they are not conscious of their diets as "diets." The diets are, as it were, culturally "natural," and cultural diets are based on foods, not nutrients.

Interventionist diets and fad diets are often based not on foods but on nutrients, or rather on three very broad categories of nutrients: fats, carbohydrates, and proteins.

Low-fat gurus like Dr. Dean Ornish want you to live as if there were no foods, just carbohydrates, proteins, and fats. And he wants you to eliminate the fats.

High-fat fad doctors like Dr. Robert Atkins also want you to forget about food. Once again it's carbohydrates, proteins, and fats, but he wants you to eliminate the carbohydrates.

Interesting ideas, but they face one little problem: Never at any time or place in human history have people lived on carbohydrates, proteins, or fats. They don't shop for them; they don't grow or raise them; they don't cook with them or trade recipes for them; and they don't celebrate Thanksgiving, Passover, or Christmas with them.

The Old Ways Preservation and Exchange Trust is an organization dedicated to preserving the wisdom of culturally based diets. Commenting on the absurdity of nutrient-focused ways of eating, Dun Gifford, Old Ways founder and president, is fond of pointing out, "There is no carbohydrate aisle at the supermarket."

People live on and with foods. People love food. And any diet that doesn't incorporate these fundamental and very human facts is bound to fail.

A Reverence for Food

While living in Rome from 1977 to 1980, I never heard an Italian of any age, male or female, talk about dieting. They had no fear of food, whether it contained fats or carbohydrates. They ate well, without guilt, until they were full, and then stopped. And when it was time to eat again, they ate with the same gusto.

They never talked about calories, or fat, or carbohydrates, or weight loss. But they did talk about food, all the time. They did not talk fearfully, but critically. Was it good food or bad food? Was it well prepared or poorly prepared? Their appreciation and criticism grew out of a reverence and love for food. Despite their disregard for fat grams, Zones, or other fad diets, the Italian people are thin by American standards. There are, of course, fat Italians—and Greeks, Spaniards, French, Lebanese, and Tunisians—but Mediterranean obesity rates are far lower than those of America.

The problem with low-fat diets is that people adopt them with all the eagerness of a long-overdue penance.

But there is another way. There is a diet, which we will explain in this book, that is not meant as a temporary, unnatural interruption in your life, but as a permanent enhancement of it. It's a diet meant to become a natural—and enjoyable—part of your lifestyle. It is neither high in fat nor low in fat. Most of the fat in this "Mediterranean diet" is fat that is positively good for you—namely, olive oil.

In our studies, real-life people who use the Mediterranean philosophy of eating are happier with their food, feel great, and can lose weight at an average of 1.5 pounds a week, a healthy pace.

Here are two notes we received from a Brown University employee enrolled in the diet study we did for this book. The first note is from the summer, when she was in the early stages of the diet, and the second is from December 1998, after she'd made the diet a regular part of her life.

> In my previous reply I forgot to include my thoughts on how this diet compares to those I tried in the past. In my opinion it is far superior. As I may have reported, my only previous diet experience was Weight Watchers.... Fats were limited.... I often felt hungry after eating all the food that was allowed for the day. I think I ate cottage cheese and lettuce for most of the five years.... I just got tired of doing this, resumed my old eating habits, and regained my lost weight and steadily added more weight.
>
> The Mediterranean diet gives me a whole new way of looking at meals. They are very easy to prepare (usually less than a half hour from preparation to table), and I feel as if I'm eating nouveau cuisine restaurant meals in my own home. I am never hungry between meals. I usually eat out once or twice a week, but I try to keep

my portion size similar to those I eat at home and I am still losing weight, so I must be doing it right.

I am so glad that I came to your lectures and volunteered for this study. I feel that I am really in control of my weight. I go in for my annual check-up next week. My primary care physician will be pleased that I have lost weight and plan to lose more.

Six months later Dr. Flynn received this e-mail from the enrollee:

> I just wanted to thank you for the Mediterranean diet study you did last spring. I was a participant and have made lifestyle changes that have had a great effect on my health and outlook. Since the study ended in July, I have lost an additional 10 pounds, making a total weight loss of 26 pounds. (This is the first year I have actually lost weight between Thanksgiving and Christmas!) My blood pressure has gone from borderline high (150/90) to normal 130/80, my cholesterol level has gone from 258 to 205, and my HDL level has gone from 57 to 61. I hadn't had previous tests for triglycerides and LDL, but this year's results were triglycerides 124 and LDL 119. I am grateful to you for having the brown bag lectures and proposing the study. I never could have accomplished this on my own.

So you can—and should—consume some fat to lose weight. As we'll see, people who go on low-fat diets fail miserably over the long term. Worse yet, many people who fail to lose weight on low-

fat diets can actually worsen their cholesterol and triglyceride levels. Further, they can deprive themselves of nutrients that might
be useful in reducing certain cancer risks.

The bottom line is, you can enjoy good food, *and* lose weight,
and improve your health. In the pages that follow, we'll show you
how.

4 Cancer, Fat, and Low-Fat Diets

For years the National Cancer Institute (NCI) and the U.S. government have been pushing low-fat diets as a way to fight cancer. But there is no conclusive evidence that low-fat diets prevent cancer. Yet there is evidence that the right fats in your diet may help prevent cancer. Cutting out the good fats could actually be dangerous.

In the NCI's "Action Guide for Healthy Eating" brochure, for instance, one theme that appears on almost every page is the need to reduce fat consumption. The NCI bemoans the fact that Americans are still eating diets containing 34 percent fat and have not yet reached the "magic" 30 percent goal. The NCI gives detailed instructions on how to calculate fat grams and specifically recommends that you eat foods that are low in fat, such as no-fat salad dressings. It seems that as far as the NCI is concerned, fat—all fat—promotes cancer. The NCI document fails to mention that certain fats can be important tools in fighting cancer.

According to this government document it's okay to eat jelly beans, gumdrops, hard candy, and angel food cake as long as not a drop of fat touches your lips. The NCI wants you to eat tons of vegetables. And that's right—vegetables are crucial cancer fighters. But it expects you to eat them steamed or raw with nothing on them, not even a drop of tasty—and very healthy—olive oil. The best they can come up with is low-fat or no-fat salad dressing.

This is unrealistic. First, most people will not eat large volumes of undressed vegetables on a continual basis. Virtually every Western culture with a cuisine rich in vegetables has developed appetizing sauces or dressings to go with them, invariably including a little fat. Depending on the *types* of fat used, those sauces can be more or less healthy. But most low-fat diet advocates, including the NCI, act as though specifying the different kinds of fats is too complicated for the American public to understand.

This oversimplification is doubly dangerous. Some fats are good for fighting cancer, and some fats may raise your risk of cancer. The cancer-inducing fats really *should* be cut out of your diet. But the NCI doesn't focus on which fats are good and which are bad.

As for the no-fat salad dressing the NCI recommends, we think you should throw yours in the trash right now. No-fat dressings may deprive you of cancer-fighting nutrients.

What Is Cancer?

Cancer comes from the Greek word for crab, because ancient physicians recognized its ability to spread, or crawl like a crab, to distant sites in the body. Lung cancer, for instance, often crawls (or metastasizes) to the brain; kidney cancer may metastasize to the lung; prostate and breast cancer tend to spread to the bones.

All cancers share one thing in common—the wildly unregulated multiplication of cells often driven by genetic abnormalities or cellular injuries. These abnormalities and injuries can be caused by agents known as *carcinogens.* One of the most famous and destructive carcinogens, for instance, is cigarette smoke.

Carcinogens don't cause cancer by themselves. There are usually multiple factors involved. The genes you inherit sometimes play a role, which may be one reason why some heavy smokers never get lung cancer and some light smokers do. Breast cancer is influenced by such unique factors as age of menarche, the number of children, use of estrogen, a family history of breast cancer, and excessive alcohol consumption. Colon cancer has a particularly strong correlation to genetics and high meat consumption. Leukemias are sometimes related to radiation exposure.

Even though different cancers are initiated and promoted by different factors, all cancers are driven by a cellular injury that causes abnormal growth. For many cancers, those injuries are initiated by biochemical reactions called *oxidation* and *free radical formation.*

You may have heard those terms before. But let's take a closer look, because oxidation and free radical formation are fundamental in the development of several diseases, including cancer, arthritis, and heart disease, and actually seem to play an important role in the aging process. Moreover, what you eat has a big impact on how much oxidation and free radical formation occurs in your body. Some diets, including some low-fat ones, can promote oxidation and may raise the risk of cancer. Other diets such as the Mediterranean diet—rich in olive oil and vegetables and with relatively little meat—can inhibit oxidation and help prevent disease.

Oxidation

All atoms are composed of electrons that orbit a central, dense mass of matter, the nucleus. The nucleus, where protons reside, carries a positive charge. The negatively charged, much smaller electrons orbit the nucleus in pairs.

When one of those electrons is lost or stolen by another atom or molecule, leaving a single, unpaired electron behind, that atom is said to have been oxidized.

Oxidation can be very damaging to cell tissue. Oxidation of metals causes rust, destroying the metal. Oxidation in our bodies can do similar damage. Not only can oxidation promote cancer, heart disease, and other diseases, aging itself may in large part be due to the accumulated damage of a lifetime of oxidation.

How does oxidation damage us? Any oxidized atom or molecule missing an electron in one of its pairs is a free radical. Certain free radicals are highly excitable: They really want their electrons back. So they try to steal electrons from other molecules. In the process they can damage various cell components such as the cell membrane; vital enzymes; mitochondria, the cell's primary energy generator; and even the DNA. Oxidation can set up a chain reaction that escalates into a destructive biochemical mêlée as atoms and molecules steal electrons from each other in a desperate attempt to keep their electron pairs intact.

That's how the body "rusts."

Despite all the damage oxidation can do, it is essential to life. Whenever we convert food and oxygen to energy, we must do it through an oxidative process. If we stop the process of oxidation, we die. The key is to keep it under control.

Fortunately the body has natural mechanisms to control oxidation. This is where diet comes in. The body's natural antioxi-

The Chain Reation of Oxidation Damaging a Cell Membrane

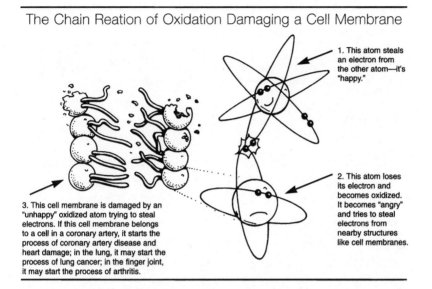

1. This atom steals an electron from the other atom—it's "happy."

2. This atom loses its electron and becomes oxidized. It becomes "angry" and tries to steal electrons from nearby structures like cell membranes.

3. This cell membrane is damaged by an "unhappy" oxidized atom trying to steal electrons. If this cell membrane belongs to a cell in a coronary artery, it starts the process of coronary artery disease and heart damage; in the lung, it may start the process of lung cancer; in the finger joint, it may start the process of arthritis.

dant defenses can be bolstered by eating foods rich in antioxidants, substances that control oxidation. Fruits and vegetables are very high in antioxidants. So are olive oil and red wine. Strong scientific evidence suggests a diet rich in antioxidants helps prevent disease and prolong life. That's probably why the people from Crete, Greece, Spain, southern France, and southern Italy, who eat a diet rich in plants, olive oil, and red wine, are among the longest-living people in the world.

Four Fats and Cancer

The fats that are most likely to promote cancer are those that are most easily oxidized. And which fats are most easily oxidized? You'll be surprised.

Why Do You Think They Call Them Saturated Fats?

For may have been hearing about saturated, polyunsaturated, and monounsaturated fats and wondering what it all really means. It comes down to how much hydrogen they hold.

When Oxygen Gets Jilted

Oxidation is about love. The love of electrons. Some atoms and molecules can endure the loss of their electrons, while others don't handle it well. Oxygen just can't bear it. Oxygen is a romantic particle. An oxygen particle that gives up an electron is called a singlet. Oxygen doesn't like to be a singlet. It would much rather have its electrons paired up so it can live happily ever after. But when the electron couple living in its outermost orbit breaks up, oxygen becomes depressed, angry, and violent. In short, it behaves radically and can do a lot of damage to the other atoms and molecules around it. There is no point in trying to console or comfort a jilted oxygen atom. It just won't be happy until it gets its electron back. That's the way love is.

Some molecules tolerate such romantic losses much better. These philosophical types usually don't become angry or violent when they lose electrons, so they can safely donate electrons to hot-tempered radicals like oxygen and calm them down. The generous compounds that exhibit this most unselfish form of love are called antioxidants.

Saturated fats are completely saturated with hydrogen. They are usually solid at room temperature, and are most commonly found in animal fat. Red meat is high in saturated fat. So are whole milk and butter. Saturated fats have a bad reputation. They are notorious for their ability to raise cholesterol and thereby promote heart disease.

But if you guessed that saturated fats oxidized easily and were therefore likely to promote cancer you'd be wrong. Don't feel bad; most physicians don't know that either. When we surveyed a group of physicians we found that 41 percent mistakenly believed saturated fats were the most easily oxidized and most likely to cause cancer.

Because saturated fats are loaded with hydrogen, they have no double bonds. The more double bonds fats have, the more likely they are to oxidize. With no double bonds saturated fats resist oxi-

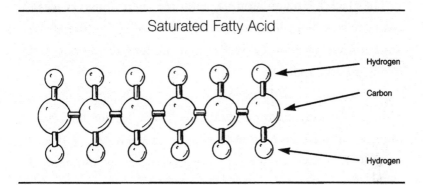

Saturated Fatty Acid

Hydrogen

Carbon

Hydrogen

dation, and so, despite some controversy over colon cancer that we will explore, much of the evidence suggests that saturated fats do not cause cancer.

Problems with Polyunsaturated Fats

Of all fats, polyunsaturated fats are most easily oxidized. Their tendency to oxidize is dramatically increased when they are heated for cooking. Experiments in animals suggest that polyunsaturated fats are more likely to promote cancer. Examples of oils with large amounts of polyunsaturated fats are corn oil, soybean oil, safflower oil, sunflower oil, cottonseed oil, and most margarines. It is the ultimate nutritional irony that these fats, which are recommended by the government and leading health agencies as heart-healthy substitutes for saturated fats, may increase your risk of cancer. We are now learning that they may also be much less desirable in heart disease prevention than the "experts" once thought.

Polyunsaturated fats (fats that are not completely saturated with hydrogen) are extracted mostly from the seeds or kernels of plants and, unlike saturated fats, are liquid at room temperature.

They lack hydrogen atoms at multiple (hence *poly*) places. At each site lacking hydrogens they have double bonds, thereby creating a predisposition to oxidize and produce dangerous, DNA-damaging free radicals.

In addition to oxidizing easily, there may be other problems with specific polyunsaturated fats. For example, linoleic acid, an omega-6 fatty acid, is used by the body to make hormone-like substances. Excessive amounts of omega-6 fats may stimulate the

Polyunsaturated Fatty Acid

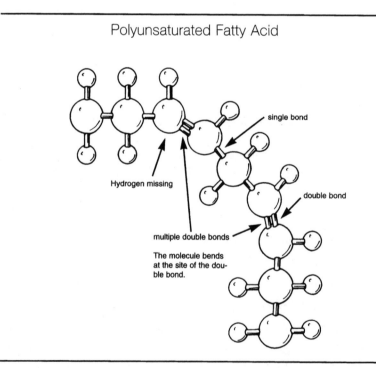

single bond

Hydrogen missing

double bond

multiple double bonds

The molecule bends at the site of the double bond.

growth of hormone-sensitive tumors such as breast, uterine, and prostate cancers.

However, as is often the case with nutrition and health, the case against polyunsaturated fats is not open and shut. Unlike saturated and monounsaturated fats, the body can't manufacture polyunsaturated fats. You need to eat a tiny amount of polyunsaturated fat so that your body can make important hormone-like substances called prostaglandins. Polyunsaturated fats can also lower LDL cholesterol and may impart healthy fluidity to cell membranes.

There is even a polyunsaturated fat that, for complicated reasons, seems positively good for you. This fat, called alpha-linolenic acid or omega-3 fatty acid, is the active ingredient in fish oil and whale blubber that probably helps keep the Japanese and the Eskimos so healthy. Famous for their role in preventing heart disease, omega-3 fatty acids seem to have cancer-fighting properties as well. Other sources of omega-3 fatty acids include walnuts and canola oil.

Trans Fats—Partially Hydrogenated and Dangerous

Ever look at the nutritional information on a box of Snackwell cookies or a Healthy Choice dinner and see the words "partially hydrogenated fats"? If you are like most people, you probably don't know what they are. Partially hydrogenated fats are unsaturated fats that have had hydrogen artificially added back to them.

Manufacturers add hydrogen to make liquid unsaturated fats more solid and easier to work with. This also increases the shelf life of these mass-produced products. Regardless of the reason, these fats, also called trans fats, are bad for you. Very bad. While not strongly associated with cancer, a high level of trans fats in the diet can dramatically increase the risk of heart disease—by 80 percent in one study. The largest doses of trans fats are in fast foods—especially french fries. Other foods like Snackwells, and lots of

---

Trans Fatty Acid

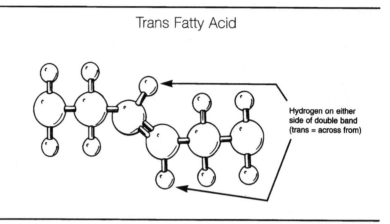

Hydrogen on either side of double band (trans = across from)

---

other baked products, have miniscule amounts, but when you add them up it may mean bad news for your heart.

The Magnificent Monounsaturated Fats

Finally we get to the real heroes in this story—monounsaturated fats. Because of their structure (one double bond), monounsaturated fats enjoy the benefits of both saturated and polyunsaturated fats and none of the drawbacks. Like saturated fats, they are highly resistant to oxidation and so won't generate a lot of cancer-causing free radicals. And like polyunsaturated fats, they can lower cholesterol and may give a healthy fluidity to cell membranes when incorporated into their structure.

The best source of monounsaturated fat is olive oil. The second-best source is canola oil. Olive oil is about 74 percent monounsaturated fat. But people sometimes forget that olive oil contains other things besides monounsaturated fat. It contains hundreds, perhaps thousands of phytochemicals, including vitamin E. So

Monos in Meat

Even though you can find monounsaturated fats (monos) in many sources, such as meat, we say olive oil is the *best* source of monos. Meat is definitely not a good source of monos because meat carries with it a lot of unfavorable nutritional baggage. It has lots of cholesterol-raising saturated fat and often a whole host of potential carcinogens. To make matters worse, meat supplies no antioxidants or phytochemicals to counteract the effects of the carcinogens it carries. The presence of monos in meat sometimes creates confusion. Monos sometimes unfairly get blamed for the damage done by the other culprits in meat.

Monounsaturated Fatty Acid

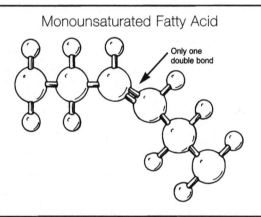

Only one double bond

monounsaturated fats not only resist oxidation, they also carry a whole supply of phytochemicals and antioxidants, giving you a double dose of antioxidant protection. If oxidation causes the body to "rust," then olive oil is the body's Rustoleum.

Not only does olive oil not cause cancer or heart disease, there is very good evidence that olive oil helps prevent these chronic diseases. Much of that evidence will be presented in this book.

You should, as much as possible, replace the saturated and polyunsaturated fats in your diet with olive oil. Ignore fat phobes like Dr. Dean Ornish who tell you that you must never partake of this delicious oil. You're not obliged to drink a cup each morning, as some Cretan centenarians are known to do, but a little bit every day is a good idea if you want to live a long and healthy life.

To say fat causes cancer is terribly misleading. It is clear that while certain kinds of fats such as polyunsaturated fats may predispose one to certain cancers, saturated fats probably play a negligible role. On the other hand, olive oil, which is rich in monounsaturated fats, may be positively beneficial in reducing cancer risks. Its benefit derives partly from its resistance to oxida-

Fatty Acid Content of Oils and Fats

	% MONO-UNSATURATED FAT	% POLY-UNSATURATED FAT, LINOLEIC ACID (N-6)	% POLY-UNSATURATED FAT, LINOLENIC ACID (N-3)	% SAT-URATED FAT
OILS:				
olive	74	8	1	14
canola	59	20	9	7
peanut	46	32	0	17
sesame	40	41	<1	14
soybean	23	51	7	14
corn	24	58	1	13
cottonseed	18	52	<1	26
safflower	12	74	<1	9
FATS:				
butter	23	2	1	51
hydrogenated soybean*	43	35	3	15
shortening*	51	14	1	31

*used in commercial products and baked goods

Eating Polyester Is Bad for Your Health

One of the worst things about the 1970s were polyester leisure suits. Well, "it's baaack." Not leisure suits—polyester. This time it's in the form of a fat substitute called olestra, or Olean. Olestra is actually a sucrose polyester, and if there is anything worse than wearing polyester, it's eating it.

The most publicized problem with olestra is its reported tendency to cause diarrhea. (Diarrhea may be a blessing in this case, because it would likely make you avoid the stuff.) But the biggest health problem with olestra is its ability to lower carotene levels, by 15 to 30 percent according to some conservative estimates.

Dr. Meir Stamfer of the Harvard School of Public Health estimates that just a 10 percent reduction in blood carotenes could yield 7,500 extra cases of lung cancer, 10,000 extra cases of prostate cancer, and 11,000 extra cases of heart disease per year. It's bad enough that olestra is in nonfat snack foods—if it ever gets into salad dressing, it may create a national carotene crisis, and those estimates may skyrocket. But despite its cancer- and disease-promoting potential, olestra, like many low- and nonfat food products, hides under a mantle of health created by nonfat fanaticism and cheerfully perpetuated by companies raking in fat wads of dough.

tion and partly from the supply of phytochemicals and antioxidants that the olive so generously imparts to the oil. But there are other reasons why olive oil may help prevent cancer, and these have to do with olive oil's special relationship with vegetables and carotenes.

Carotenes, Fat, and Cancer Prevention

Plants can't move. They're planted. They can't run from predators, flee epidemics, avoid carcinogenic toxins, or seek shelter from the relentless DNA-damaging rays of the sun. They must stand and fight, and one of the most potent weapons they have at their disposal are the hundreds of thousands of phytochemicals that plants produce. Literally translated, "phytochemical" means "chemicals found in plants." When we eat plants we consume these newly discovered protective compounds.

Carotenoids are just one large class of the many different kinds of phytochemicals. Yet there are at least five hundred different carotenoids, and each of these, in turn, has many different forms called isomers.

Carotenoids can be divided into carotenes and oxycarotenoids. Beta-carotene is the best-known carotene because it was one of the first that researchers were able to identify and measure in the blood, but there are many other carotenes as well.

Carotenes are best known for their impressive antioxidant capabilities. But there may be other ways in which these phytochemicals may inhibit the development of cancer. For instance, there is evidence that cancerous cells divide in an uncontrolled fashion because they fail to communicate properly with normal cells that could otherwise slow down their replication. At least one study has shown that carotenes may help normal cells communicate with potentially cancerous cells and thereby inhibit the replication of cancer cells. Other research suggests that carotenes encourage cells to mature and develop specific, specialized functions. Such mature cells are much less likely to become cancerous. It seems that besides being antioxidants, carotenes have multiple mechanisms by which they can potentially prevent cancer.

But carotenes have another property that distinguishes them from other phytochemicals—they are lipophilic, or fat loving. That means if you don't eat any fat within a few hours of consuming carotenes, you won't absorb them.

Translation: Use no-fat salad dressing on you're salad and you're likely to flush most of the cancer-preventing carotenes in that salad right down the toilet.

Of course you don't want to put cholesterol-raising saturated fat on your salad. Polyunsaturated fats are also out, as are the partially hydrogenated fats in some low-fat salad dressings. What are you left with? Olive oil:

For many reasons olive oil is the ideal fat for people interested in reducing their risk of cancer. Olive oil

- is rich in oxidation-resistant monounsaturated fat,

- carries its own supply of cancer-fighting phytochemicals and antioxidants,

- tastes good and promotes greater consumption of cancer-fighting vegetables, and

- permits the absorption of cancer-fighting carotenes.

Olive oil is not an abstract macronutrient like fat, carbohydrates, or protein. It is a real food, and it is the foundation for a spectrum of culturally evolved cuisines in the Mediterranean basin—cuisines that have proven their value in reducing the risks of cancer. Also, olive oil's relationship to vegetables is straightforward. It makes them delicious, so we will eat more of them. And the more vegetables we eat, the less likely we are to develop cancer.

It is very hard to believe that in the face of these advantages the

Vitamin E, Fat, and Cancer

Vitamin E is the miracle pill of the new millennium. It's being used in experiments for a broad spectrum of diseases, from cancer to heart disease to arthritis to Alzheimer's. Oxidation plays a role in all these diseases, and vitamin E is a powerful antioxidant. A number of studies have shown that vitamin E helps prevent cancer and heart disease. However, nature hasn't endowed any single plant with particularly high doses of vitamin E. There is some in kale, collard greens, nuts, and wheat germ. The most plentiful natural sources are certain plant oils. Polyunsaturated fats such as safflower oil and soybean oil contain relatively generous amounts of vitamin E. Unfortunately these fats oxidize easily, creating dangerous free radicals. Consequently a significant amount of the vitamin E in these

NCI would recommend low-fat and no-fat salad dressing over healthy olive oil. It seems as though the NCI has also been sucked in by the low-fat lie.

Colon Cancer and Fat—Accomplice or Innocent Bystander?

Colon cancer is the fourth-leading cause of cancer deaths in the United States after lung, breast, and prostate cancer. Colon cancer is also a principal source of the low-fat fallacy that fats in general, and saturated fats in particular, cause cancer.

At first it looks like a pretty strong case against fat. Population studies reveal that, with two notable exceptions (Greece and Finland), countries with the greatest fat-consumption get the most colon cancer. But on closer examination it seems more likely that fats, particularly saturated and monounsaturated fats, are getting a bad rap merely for the company they keep.

polyunsaturated oils is consumed to suppress the free radicals these oils create in the first place. Not very efficient.

Once again olive oil comes to the rescue. It contains a healthy dose of vitamin E, and because olive oil doesn't oxidize easily, the vitamin E it contains stands ready to fight free radicals that are generated from other sources. And unlike in other oils, virtually all the vitamin E in olive oil is in the most potent form, called alpha tocopherol.

At least one study has shown that a very-low-fat diet decreases the body's levels of vitamin E. The bottom line is that olive oil is one of the best natural sources of vitamin E. If you are on a low-fat diet that forbids nuts and olive oil, you will be depriving yourself of important sources of vitamin E. You can take supplements if you like, but they are a poor substitute for a healthy diet.

It is well known that most dietary saturated fat comes from meat. But it is not well known that meat also contains monounsaturated fat. In fact in the U.S., where olive oil is not widely consumed, Americans get most of their monounsaturated fat from meat. Unfortunately it does them little good because of the other, less healthy substances in meat.

Meat is full of potential carcinogens, such as iron. Just as the iron outside the body is prone to oxidize and rust, iron inside the body is prone to oxidation and free radical formation. Processed meats like bacon have carcinogens called nitrosamines. And when meat or fish is cooked so that it is seared and browned, it produces other carcinogens called heterocyclic amines. About twenty different heterocyclic amines have been identified in cooked meat, and they are known to promote colon, breast, pancreatic, and prostate cancer in rats.

Both saturated fats and monounsaturated fats are probably

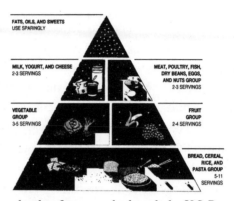

While the NCI pushes low fat across the board, the U.S. Department of Agriculture pushes meat and everything in it—saturated fat and all the potential carcinogens. In the USDA food pyramid, which was developed under the influence of the meat lobby, meat appears close to the middle of the pyramid. It is placed with beans, nuts, and fish, giving the impression that it is just as healthy. Worse, it is accompanied by a written directive to consume two or three servings per day. While this may be great for the beef industry and Burger King, it's disastrous for you and your children. Yet this is the pyramid that hangs in classrooms and doctors' offices.

innocent bystanders getting a bad rap because they hang out with the carcinogens in top sirloin and fast-food cheeseburgers and hamburgers.

On the other hand there is evidence that olive oil, a positively good fat, may offer protection against the carcinogens in meat. Not only does the monounsaturated fat in olive oil resist oxidation, the oil is also full of the olive's phytochemicals, which may protect against some of the carcinogens in meat. For instance, it seems that the cancer-causing nitrosamines must form links with other compounds in our digestive tracts before they can do their dirty work. However, it has recently been discovered that olive oil contains certain phytochemicals (e.g., ferulic acid and chlorogenic acid) that can prevent these compounds from linking together. Olive oil has still other phytochemicals (caffeic acid and luteolin) that inhibit the formation of heterocyclic amines when meat or fish is seared.

Eat the Plant, Not the Pill

There are hundreds of thousands of phytochemicals out there, and that's one reason eating a rich variety of fruits, vegetables, nuts, and beans is so important. Sure you can get beta-carotene in a pill, but you'd still be missing out on thousands of other phytochemicals. This is an important reason why people who eat a wide variety of fruits and vegetables, such as the Mediterraneans, get cancer less frequently. One very disturbing study from Finland shows that smokers who took beta-carotene pills had higher rates of lung cancer. Solitary beta-carotene without the reinforcements of thousands of other phytochemicals working together seemed to make matters worse in this study. When it comes to your diet, you should eat as many different plants as possible. The Mediterranean diet, which has a variety of plant-based foods, offers an extraordinary pharmacopoeia of phytochemicals.

When you sift through all the evidence, you come up with something like this: It is probably the carcinogens in meat, not saturated or monounsaturated fats, that cause diet-related colon cancer. Although in population studies fat intake of all kinds seems to be related to colon cancer, this relationship breaks down in countries consuming large amounts of olive oil (Greece) or high amounts of fiber (Finland).

The Mediterranean diet, low in meat, rich in fiber, and steeped in olive oil, offers ideal protection against colon cancer. Instead of telling us to use no-fat salad dressing and offering abstract advice about cutting our dietary fat to some arbitrary percentage, the NCI should be telling us to eat like Mediterraneans.

Breast Cancer and Fat

Many researchers have argued that dietary fat promotes breast cancer, and the NCI documents echo that belief. As with colon cancer, impressive graphs show that as you consume more fat you are more likely to get breast cancer. But once again these graphs can be misleading. A recent study showed that eating well-done meat is associated with breast cancer. Once again the fat in the meat may be an innocent bystander while other carcinogens, like heterocyclic amines formed by cooking meat, do the damage.

In very large studies of women living in the United States and Europe, there has been no significant correlation between breast cancer and the amount of fat women ate. In Greece, Italy, and Spain, where the consumption of fat in the form of olive oil is very high, the rates of breast cancer are lower than in other Western countries where women eat less fat.

In animals the fats that do seem to promote breast cancer are the polyunsaturated fats—particularly the omega-6 fats found in corn, safflower, and soybean oils that we are encouraged to eat because they can lower cholesterol. This tendency may be related both to the ability of polyunsaturated fats to oxidize and their ability to stimulate hormone-sensitive tumors.

On the other hand, in five recent studies (the Nurses' Health Study and other studies carried out in Spain, Greece, Italy, and Sweden) it was demonstrated that diets rich in olive oil and monounsaturated fats were associated with lower rates of breast cancer. The most recent study was in Sweden. In this study it was also quite clear that saturated fat did not appear to be associated with breast cancer, but easily oxidized polyunsaturated fats did raise the risk of breast cancer, just as they did in animal experiments.

The evidence shows that breast cancer is more likely to be related

Dressed to Kill: Cancer and Nonfat Salad Dressing

You've finally resolved to eat better, but you just can't accept that olive oil, a fat, could possibly be good for you. So as the National Cancer Institute has suggested, you went out to the store and bought a few bottles of nonfat salad dressing and every fruit and vegetable in sight. Now you're on the second week of your low-fat diet, you've managed to eat a salad every day, and you're feeling proud. After all, the salad is full of arugula, broccoli bits, carrots, and other high-fiber, carotene-rich foods. And you've consumed this bounty of healthy food with nary a single gram of fat because you have dutifully obeyed the no-fat mantra and used only nonfat salad dressing. Low-cal, low-fat, and supernutritious—it doesn't get any better than this for a low-fat dieter, right? Wrong.

By cutting the fat out of your salad dressing, you may have cheated yourself out of some of the most significant health benefits that salad has to offer. One of the best-kept secrets about carotenes—plant-derived, cancer-fighting phytochemicals—is that you need a little fat to absorb them. Eat no fat and the carotene passes through your system and, quite literally, goes down the drain. You can rest assured that the manufacturers of nonfat salad dressing aren't going to share this secret with you.

to obesity (how fat you are) than fat intake (how much fat you eat). One reason may be that obese women produce more estrogen, which stimulates the growth of hormone-sensitive breast tumors. Of course fat phobes will argue that dietary fat makes you obese. But they are on shaky ground when they make that assumption. Dr. Walter Willet reviewed dietary fat and breast cancer in his book *Nutritional Epidemiology*. He concludes, "Existing data... provide little support for the hypothesis that reduction in dietary fat... will lead to substantial reductions in breast cancer in Western cultures."

Once again the key is not the quantity of fat consumed but the kind of fat. When it comes to breast cancer, indiscriminately banishing fat and blindly adhering to low-fat diets will deprive women of the protective effects that seem to be associated with monounsaturated fats like olive oil and canola oil. The NCI has funded wonderful research in the fight against cancer, but it just can't seem to shake the low-fat lie.

How Pizza Might Prevent Prostate Cancer

New evidence suggests that a particularly potent carotene called lycopene plays an important role in the prevention of prostate cancer, and fat plays a critical role in the story. Lycopene is found in tomatoes but, like other carotenes, you don't absorb it well without a little fat. It has been shown that men who eat more marinara sauce—the kind that goes on pizza and pasta—have lower rates of prostate cancer. Of course, when properly prepared, marinara sauce always has a little olive oil. Cut out the olive oil, and the tomato sauce loses much of its preventive power. Without a little fat, the lycopene in tomatoes is as useless as a Ferrari without gas. So all those fat-phobic recipes for tomato sauce are not only tasteless, but they are downright wasteful.

Lung Cancer

Lung cancer is the leading cause of cancer deaths in the United States, followed by breast cancer for women and prostate cancer for men. No other factor correlates with lung cancer as closely as smoking. Fat has not been associated with lung cancer, and most people don't even associate lung cancer with diet. Yet researchers who work in the field have long observed that there is an inverse relationship between yellow and green vegetables, carotenes, and lung cancer; that is, people who consume more yellow and green vegetables and have higher levels of carotenes have lower rates of lung cancer.

As you now know, fats like olive oil are very important for the absorption of carotenes. And as Dr. Antonia Trichopoulou of the University of Athens has pointed out, olive oil makes green vegetables palatable. It is not unreasonable to propose that olive oil and a diet rich in plant-based carotenes and other phytochemicals play a large role in preventing lung cancer in Mediterranean countries. Otherwise it would be very hard to explain why Mediterraneans who are heavy smokers enjoy such low rates of lung cancer. Something is protecting them.

Deviating from Dogma

It's hard to know why the NCI has so largely ignored the arguments supporting the importance of monounsaturated fats, olive oil, and the Mediterranean diet in cancer prevention. We don't think it is lying in the literal sense, but we do suspect that it has been influenced by the ubiquity of the low-fat lie, which has prevented it from interpreting the medical literature in an objective fashion. After all everyone "knows" that fat—all fat—is bad. And so the NCI couldn't possibly write a position paper suggesting that this might not be the case. That would put the NCI at odds with the dominant dietary dogma of the day and threaten the reputation of the NCI. Best to avoid making any waves. It's certainly more comfortable.

The problem is that the dogma is not true, and the NCI's acquiescence just perpetuates the low-fat lie. By perpetuating the lie, the NCI prevents people from discovering a diet that may work for them: a diet that tastes wonderful, satisfies hunger, helps control weight, and, yes, helps prevent heart disease and cancer—the Mediterranean diet.

5 Can Low-Fat Diets Worsen Your Cholesterol?

onsider the case of Dr. Charles "Chuck" Sherman. He is forty-four years old and an outstanding pulmonologist (lung doctor). He has a lovely wife and is the father of two beautiful children. Haunted by the memory of losing his own father at an early age, he wanted to assess his risk of heart disease when he turned forty. He tested his blood for the traditional marker of cardiac risk, cholesterol. The results were not very good. His HDL, or "good cholesterol," was only 34, while his LDL, or "bad cholesterol," was 129. His triglyceride levels were elevated at 285. So Chuck did what any American living in a fat-free culture would do. He went on a low-fat diet.

Several months later, feeling justifiably proud of his dietary dedication, he had his blood lipids remeasured. To his amazement they were worse. His HDL had gone down, his LDL had barely budged, and his triglyceride level had gone up. He was shocked and mystified.

What happened? Chuck did all the right things. He did what most doctors, the American Heart Association, the National Cholesterol Education Program, Dr. Dean Ornish, and a host of food manufacturers constantly tell us to do: cut out the fat. Chuck cut the fat out of his diet, but his blood lipids did not improve. In fact they got worse. How could that be? Chuck, like most people (including physicians), heard only part of the story.

The low-fat diet has been the cornerstone of the national strategy to prevent heart disease since 1977, when the Senate Subcommittee on Nutrition and Human Needs declared it so. The low-fat diet has been adopted by the American Heart Association and the National Cholesterol Education Program as well as by physicians and dietitians across the country. It is no secret that since the Senate declared war on dietary fat, Americans have only gotten fatter. What does seem to be a secret, however, is that *low-fat diets can actually make your blood fats worse.* Eating a low-fat diet *can* lower your LDL, but a low-fat diet can also lower your levels of HDL and raise your levels of harmful triglycerides. A recent study suggests that in some people it may also convert LDL into a more dangerous type of LDL, which plays a significant role in heart disease.

Fat and Heart Disease

When we talk about heart disease, we most often mean coronary artery disease. Coronary artery disease, which generally strikes in late adulthood, has been epidemic in America and northern Europe for more than fifty years. In coronary artery disease, the blood vessels feeding the heart are diseased. Without adequate blood flow, the heart can be damaged or destroyed.

The coronary arteries lie on top of the heart and supply it with oxygen and nutrients as it constantly pumps blood out of its chambers and through the aorta to the rest of the body. Coronary artery disease occurs when the inside walls of the coronary arteries are damaged. The body heals the damage, but during the healing process a scab-like plaque forms over the injury site,

---

The Gradual Damage of Coronary Arteries Which Supply the Heart with Blood

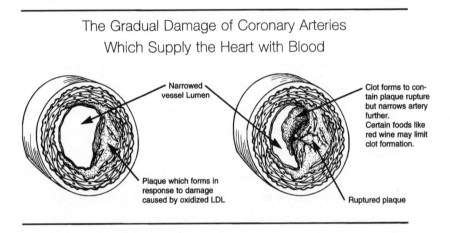

Narrowed vessel Lumen

Clot forms to contain plaque rupture but narrows artery further.
Certain foods like red wine may limit clot formation.

Plaque which forms in response to damage caused by oxidized LDL

Ruptured plaque

---

narrowing the passageway. Over the years, the cycle of injury, healing, plaque formation, and further injury continues, and the inside of the blood vessel gets narrower and narrower. Eventually the vessel gets so narrow that blood can barely get through to feed the heart. As this process, called atherosclerosis (which literally means hardening of the arteries), progresses, these vessels not only get narrower, they also get stiffer.

Normal arteries release substances such as nitric oxide or prostacylin to help them widen so they can accommodate a greater flow of blood when the heart needs it. But these stiff, plaque-lined arteries not only get dangerously narrow, they also lose the ability to expand or dilate. If the plaque suddenly ruptures, as sometimes happens, and a clot forms depriving the heart of blood, heart damage may ensue. If the damage is so severe that chunks of heart muscle die, we call it a heart attack or a myocardial infarction. If it's a very large heart attack the patient may die.

But what causes heart disease and heart attacks?

We have long known that blood cholesterol, in some way, plays a role. In fact, for thirty years blood cholesterol has ruled the world of cardiac risk. Convincing research tied blood cholesterol, a special ring-shaped fat used by the body to make hormones, to an increased risk of heart disease, and as a nation we have focused narrowly on reducing blood cholesterol. At first people did this by trying to eat less cholesterol, and many still do. Actually the cholesterol you eat has very little to do with the cholesterol that circulates in your blood, because your body makes its own. Most people can balance blood cholesterol by making less of it when they eat more cholesterol in their diet. The fat most responsible for raising cholesterol in your blood is that old devil saturated fat, which is found mostly in meat and dairy products.

Saturated Fat and Cholesterol

Starting in the 1970s, Americans were instructed to reduce saturated fat by eating low-fat diets—reducing fat across the board. They were also instructed to eat polyunsaturated fats like corn oil and margarine in lieu of saturated fats because it was discovered that polyunsaturated fats can lower total cholesterol. It was only years later that we learned that polyunsaturated fats like corn oil and soybean oil may increase the risk of other diseases because they oxidize so easily. As previously mentioned, polyunsaturated fats may promote certain cancers. In addition, margarines, as we will discuss later, have other bad fats that can worsen heart disease.

As we learned more about blood cholesterol, we discovered

Why Olive Oil?

Monounsaturated fat, the main type of fat in olive oil, lowers LDL while maintaining or raising HDL. Replacing some carbohydrates with olive oil may also suppress the increase of triglyceride levels and prevent the undesirable shift from large to small LDL in the blood. Also, olive oil resists oxidation and comes with a particularly rich supply of antioxidants. That means double protection: Less bad cholesterol in your system, and the bad cholesterol you do have is less likely to be oxidized and is, therefore, less dangerous.

that there are two different ways to carry cholesterol in the blood. The two different cholesterol carriers are high-density lipoprotein, called HDL, and low-density lipoprotein, called LDL. Elevated levels of LDL cholesterol were found to increase the risk of heart disease, while elevated levels of HDL cholesterol were found to reduce the risk of heart disease. When levels of HDL fall, the risk of heart disease goes up. It's not completely understood why this is so. One reason seems to be that HDL transports cholesterol away from the tissues and blood vessels (where it can do its damage) back to the liver, where it is safely disposed of. Another recent theory is that HDL promotes other substances that reduce the tendency of blood to clot and so make it less likely that coronary arteries will get clogged up.

As the importance of HDL in preventing heart disease was recognized, the LDL/HDL ratio was introduced. The objective was to minimize this ratio by lowering LDL as much as possible while increasing HDL. Unfortunately the dietary advice most doctors gave to lower LDL—cut out fats—also tends to lower HDL.

That's right. Low-fat diets, especially diets that replace fats with carbohydrates, reduce both types of cholesterol—good *and* bad.

Proponents of low-fat diets often dismiss this by saying that there is no evidence showing that low HDL levels are dangerous when the reduction is caused by diet. Yet, in fact, no study of the effects of low HDL on heart disease has conclusively distinguished between patients whose HDL was reduced by diet and those whose HDL was low for some other reason.

> Eighty-two percent of physicians responding to our survey did not know low-fat diets would decrease HDL cholesterol.

Almost everything we do know suggests that low HDL levels and heart disease go together like beer and pretzels. And a low-fat diet certainly can reduce your HDL.

As we shall see there are ways to get both of these blood fats moving in the right direction—up for HDL and down for LDL—but for most people a low-fat diet is *not* the answer.

Small Cholesterol, James Cagney, and Coronary Disease

Still, a low-fat diet does reduce the bad cholesterol as well as the good cholesterol. Isn't that a reasonable trade-off? Maybe not. Recent research suggests that in some people a low-fat diet can actually convert the bad cholesterol into an even worse form of bad cholesterol.

It turns out that not all LDL is alike. Some LDL particles are large, fluffy, and relatively benign. These fluffy particles do not do much damage to artery walls because they are not very good at burrowing into the walls and are more resistant to oxidation. Other LDL particles are small, prone to oxidation, and very aggressive. Two people can have the exact same cholesterol level and even the same ratio of LDL to HDL, yet one can have far more *small* LDL particles. It is these small, oxidized LDL particles that do most of the damage to our arteries.

How does the small LDL damage our arteries? Not surprisingly, as suggested above, it involves our old adversaries, oxidation and free radical formation.

One of the early events in coronary artery disease occurs when small LDL cholesterol particles undergo oxidation and burrow into the wall of the blood vessel. As previously mentioned, oxidation involves the loss of electrons, which makes the atom or molecule losing them highly agitated. The agitated LDL damages the blood vessel, creating inflammation and causing other small LDL particles to oxidize.

The body sends in white blood cells and platelets for damage control. But that can actually make the problem worse. Small LDL cholesterol particles are like Jimmy Cagney in the old gangster movies: Cagney was little, but he was very irritable. He did not deal well with authority. Small, oxidized LDL is the same way. When the white cells come in to control small, oxidized LDL, the conflict merely escalates, and inflammation spreads. Platelets, which cause blood to clot, come in and seal off microscopic damage caused by spreading inflammation, which makes matters worse because the tiny clots accumulate and contribute to further plaque formation. After years and years of damage and layer upon layer of repair, clot, and cellular debris, the passageway inside the blood vessel, called the lumen, can become quite narrow. Along the way the artery suffers from a reduced capacity to make substances that stimulate the artery to expand or dilate. These beneficial substances, prostacyclin and nitric oxide, also have the ability to prevent blood from clotting. Nitric oxide is so important

Heart, Coronary Arteries, and an Area of Blockage

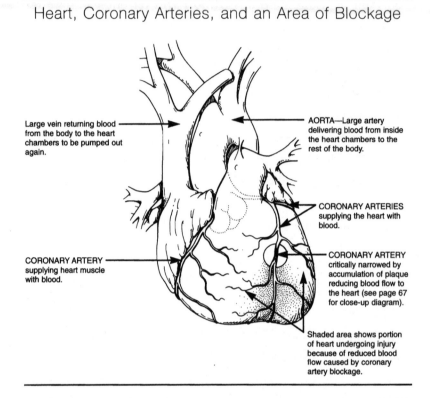

Large vein returning blood from the body to the heart chambers to be pumped out again.

AORTA—Large artery delivering blood from inside the heart chambers to the rest of the body.

CORONARY ARTERIES supplying the heart with blood.

CORONARY ARTERY supplying heart muscle with blood.

CORONARY ARTERY critically narrowed by accumulation of plaque reducing blood flow to the heart (see page 67 for close-up diagram).

Shaded area shows portion of heart undergoing injury because of reduced blood flow caused by coronary artery blockage.

that the scientists who discovered its important role in the body were awarded the Nobel Prize in 1998. As we shall see later, certain foods are very valuable because of the way they affect nitric oxide and prostacyclin.

The process takes years, and it goes something like this:

1) Small LDL oxidizes, then burrows into artery walls.

2) Inflammation.

3) More oxidation.

4) Blood clotting.

5) Plaque formation.

6) Reduced nitric oxide.

7) Stiff vessels.

8) More clotting.

9) Blockage.

10) Heart attack.

That's the sequence. And the oxidation of small LDL starts the whole ball rolling.

Low-Fat Diets, Small LDL, and Triglycerides

So, how do we end up with lots of small LDL? Well, diet can have a significant influence on cholesterol's particle size and propensity to oxidize. HDL and triglycerides have a seesaw relationship. As triglyceride levels go up, HDL levels go down. But triglycerides are also related to small LDL. As triglyceride levels go up, small LDL levels also go up. There is strong evidence that in some people diets low in fat and high in carbohydrates, such as those recommended by the National Cholesterol Education Program, actually promote the development of the small, dense LDL particles that are more likely to burrow into blood vessels and oxidize.

In a recent experiment Dr. Ron Krauss, who is also the former chairman of the nutrition committee of the American Heart Association, put 105 men on a low-fat American Heart Association-type diet. He found that in many of these men, HDL levels went down and triglyceride levels went up, just as many studies have shown in the past. But most of those studies were done before we knew about large and small LDL. Krauss found that 34 percent of the men on a low-fat, high-carbohydrate diet also shifted their LDL particle type from the large, fluffy, benign kind to the small, aggressive kind. This pattern of low HDL levels and elevated levels of triglycerides and small LDL is called pattern B. Pattern B is associated with an increased risk of heart disease. Several other studies have shown similar results.

When asked what size cholesterol was most dangerous to arteries, 77 percent of physicians responding to our survey did not know that small LDL was most dangerous.

What will happen to the men who shifted to small LDL cholesterol if they continue on a low-fat diet is unclear. It depends in part on what their genes are like and whether they exercise or lose weight. It also depends on whether they eat a diet rich in antioxidants. But a prudent person would want to minimize risk as much as possible. It makes more sense to choose a diet that will preserve HDL while lowering levels of triglycerides and small LDL. Eating a little more of the right kind of fat, like olive oil, and fewer carbohydrates can prevent these kinds of shifts.

The Critical Lower Boundary of Fat

The low-fat diet that Dr. Krauss used derived about 25 percent of its calories from fat. The 25-percent-fat mark appears to be a critical lower boundary. At that point total LDL levels tend to stop going down, and the LDL you do have gets smaller as triglyceride levels go up. But many so-called low-fat diets are much more extreme and may produce even more powerful and undesirable effects on your blood fats.

In fact, one big problem with all the low-fat propaganda is that in the midst of all the hysteria it is almost impossible to come up with a common definition of a low-fat diet. The average American consumes only 34 percent of calories from fat, down from almost 40 percent a few decades ago. The American Heart Association recommends a diet of not more than 30 percent of calories from fat. Initially, it did not give any lower limit, the implication being the less fat, the better. Only in the summer of 1998 did the American Heart Association finally define a very-low-fat diet as less than 15 percent of calories from fat. How low should you go?

We recently polled several hundred physicians and asked them to define a low-fat diet. They provided a broad range of answers that illustrates the confusion over what low-fat means. Sixty percent felt that a "low-fat diet" was a diet in which less than 20 percent of calories come from fat. This is far lower and far more difficult to achieve than the more reasonable 30 percent American Heart Association threshold quoted above. But for many, even this wasn't low enough. Forty percent of physicians thought that a low-fat diet was less than 15 percent fat—an extremely difficult goal in American society and well below the threshold where levels of dangerous triglycerides and small LDL rise if there is no weight loss or exercise.

Some low-fat proponents like Dr. Dean Ornish would set the bar even lower. He recommends getting less than 10 percent of all calories from fat sources. This would require eliminating every detectable gram of fat from your diet (sometimes he grudgingly allows a tiny dose of fish oil or flaxseed oil).

In short, many Americans have become convinced that it is imperative for them to pursue extremely low-fat diets, with virtually no warning about the possible harm of doing so. We have seen several dangers so far. Very-low-fat diets may impair your absorption of vital cancer-fighting nutrients called carotenes. A low-fat, high-carbohydrate diet can reduce levels of good HDL. And while that diet can also reduce levels of bad LDL, in some people it can make the LDL smaller, more dangerous, and more aggressive.

Now let's look at the blood fat everyone ignores, but is at the heart of the matter: triglycerides.

6 The Danger Your Doctor Doesn't Talk About

Even if you had your annual physical within the past month, you probably can't quote your triglyceride measurement unless it was off the charts. That's not surprising. Many physicians overlook triglycerides. Your doctor may not have even mentioned them to you. After telling you your cholesterol level he or she may have dismissed your triglycerides with the usual catchall phrase "And all your other lab tests were normal."

Your doctor probably doesn't pay much attention to triglycerides for the same reason you don't: Triglycerides have not gotten nearly as much publicity as cholesterol. When the National Cholesterol Education Program encouraged all Americans to "know their number," it wasn't talking about triglycerides. Triglycerides are the forgotten risk factor in heart disease.

In the past some experts doubted the significance of triglycerides unless the levels were sky-high or diabetes was present. In fact as recently as 1996 the American College of Physicians didn't even recommend measuring a patient's triglyceride levels on an initial screening for risk of heart disease.

The government-sponsored Natural Cholesterol Education Program says that fasting triglyceride levels up to 200 milligrams per deciliter (mg/dl) are normal, 200 to 400 mg/dl are mildly to moderately elevated, and over 400 mg/dl are very elevated. Consequently, many physicians don't get excited until they see triglyceride levels over 400, if they check them at all.

Dismissing triglycerides is risky. Even triglyceride levels far below the officially sanctioned limit of 200 are strongly associated with increased cardiac risk.

For instance, Dr. Jorgen Jeppesen and his colleagues followed 2,906 men for eight years in the Copenhagen Heart Study and found that triglycerides were an independent risk factor for coronary artery disease. Their results, published in 1998, demonstrated that, even after taking into account other risk factors like LDL and HDL cholesterol, risk increased as the triglyceride levels increased. Furthermore, they showed that even triglyceride levels currently considered in the normal range—that is, less than 200—are associated with increased risk.

In another recent study of heart patients conducted by Dr. Michael Miller at the University of Maryland Medical Center, triglyceride levels as low as 100 presented significantly increased risk compared with levels below 100.

Triglycerides: How to Keep Your Levels Down

In one sense triglycerides are very simple: They are the fats that supply your body with energy. Cholesterol, the other blood fat, is not an energy source. That's why your fat cells store fat in triglyceride form—so you can use the energy later.

Like cholesterol and all other fats, triglycerides are not soluble in water. And so, to travel through our blood they must have a water-soluble transport vessel (lipoprotein), just like cholesterol does.

Most triglycerides travel in a vessel called VLDL (very low density lipoprotein), but some triglycerides are carried by LDL. LDLs that carry more triglycerides are more likely to become small, mean LDL, the dangerous kind. How? Well, when you have a high fasting level of triglycerides in your blood, your LDL ends up

Recommendations for Lipid and Lipoprotein Levels

When getting a physical examination ask your physician for your total cholesterol level, LDL-cholesterol level, HDL-cholesterol level, and triglyceride level. You need to fast for 12 hours before your exam to receive an accurate value for triglycerides (this is your "fasting" triglyceride level).

NCEP recommendations	Comments	Our suggested Goals
Total Cholesterol: less than 200	This is reasonable, and 200 is a round number that's easy to remember. In the Seven Country Study, the heart-healthiest men had total cholesterol levels of about 200 mg/dl and the lowest rates of heart disease. But more important than total cholesterol is the breakdown of LDL and HDL, and whether they are oxidized. A total cholesterol level of 210 or 220 is reasonable for someone without heart disease and an HDL level of 60 or 70.	about 200
LDL Cholesterol: no heart disease—less than 160; no heart disease with 2 risk factors—less than 130; heart disease—less than 100	This is controversial. Some feel that those with heart disease should be less than 100. For most that requires medication. Others feel that even those with heart disease get little added benefit from going below an LDL of 125. Once your LDL is that low it is probably more important to minimize small, oxidized LDL and to managing HDL and triglycerides. A level of 160 is probably too high.	see comments
HDL Cholesterol: greater than 35	This level is too low and it does not differentiate between men and women. For protection against coronary heart disease, men should aim for an HDL level of at least 40 mg/dl and women at least 50 mg/dl. For both men and women, the higher the HDL level, the better.	for men: 40 or higher; for women: 50 or higher
Triglycerides: less than 200	This level is too high for fasting triglycerides. When fasting triglyceride levels increase over 100 mg/dl, small LDL particles rise. When triglycerides are over 150 mg/dl often most LDL particles are small. Fasting triglycerides should be less than 100 mg/dl, but the lower the better.	less than 100

Your Fasting Triglyceride Level

Triglycerides enter your blood in two ways. One way is through ingestion. Saturated fats (from steak or butter), polyunsaturated fats (from corn oil or soybean oil), and monounsaturated fats (from olive oil) are all ingested as triglycerides. Triglycerides are simply three (tri-) chains of monounsaturated, polyunsaturated, or saturated fats linked together by a glycerol backbone.

The other way triglycerides get into the blood is through your liver, which makes and secretes them. The triglycerides from your liver are what your doctor measures. It is these triglycerides that are most often used in predicting the risk of heart disease.

To make sure only the triglycerides from the liver are measured and not the ones that come from the Egg McMuffin you had for breakfast, your doctor will ask you to fast for at least twelve hours before blood is to be drawn.

transporting more triglycerides than usual. LDL that is extra-rich in triglycerides attracts the activity of an enzyme that chops up LDL particles into even smaller LDL particles. And so more small, dangerous LDLs are born. So, the more triglycerides in the blood, the smaller the LDL gets, and the greater the risk of heart disease.

In 1992 Dr. William Castelli, former director of the famous Framingham Heart Study, found that when fasting levels of triglycerides reach 150, almost all of the LDL shifts over to the smaller size. Nonetheless, the National Cholesterol Education Program still considers triglyceride levels up to 200 to be normal.

Triglycerides and Low-Fat Diets

And what raises your fasting triglyceride level? You might think it's a high-fat diet loaded with dietary triglycerides, but it's not. It's a low-fat, high-carbohydrate diet, especially if you don't lose weight on it or if you don't exercise. Don't feel bad if you didn't know that; most doctors don't know it either.

We conducted a survey of physicians and asked the following question: What is the dietary component most likely to raise triglyceride levels? An alarming 40 percent said fat. That's simply wrong. The dietary component most likely to raise triglyceride levels is carbohydrates. And remember, when you have elevated triglyceride levels you are also more likely to have more small, easily oxidized LDL and unfavorably low HDL—that is, the dangerous pattern B described in Chapter 5.

How does a high-carbohydrate diet raise triglyceride levels? One theory relates it to insulin. A high-carbohydrate diet tends to raise insulin levels. It appears that higher insulin levels make it harder for triglycerides to get into muscle cells. This traps more triglycerides outside the cell, thereby driving blood triglyceride levels higher. On the other hand, on a lower-carbohydrate diet or with weight loss or exercise, insulin tends to fall. A lower insulin level means that triglycerides have an easier time getting into the muscle cell, where they are used for energy. This lowers blood triglyceride levels.

> When we asked doctors what would happen to someone who goes on a low-fat diet without weight loss, 63 percent did not know that triglycerides increased. When asked which diet component was most likely to raise fasting triglycerides, 50 percent did not know it was carbohydrates, and 40 percent mistakenly thought it was dietary fat.

One argument used by defenders of low-fat diets is the claim that the increase in triglycerides caused by low-fat, high-carbohy-drate diets is only temporary. They claim that the body readjusts and triglyceride levels go back to normal, even on a low-fat, high-carbohydrate diet.

Doubtful. This claim appears to be based on one study from forty years ago conducted on South African prisoners. After several months of consuming a high-carbohydrate diet, triglyceride levels that initially went up returned to normal. I think you would agree that the living conditions, caloric intake, lean body mass, and exercise levels of South African prisoners do not resemble that of sedentary Americans. The preponderance of evidence shows that when high carbohydrate diets drive up triglyceride levels, they stay up as long as the diet is continued.

The South African experiment does point out an important fact. A low-fat, high-carbohydrate diet may not raise your triglycerides if you actually lose weight on the diet or if you get lots of exercise. Unfortunately, most Americans on low-fat diets do neither.

Triglycerides and the National Cholesterol Education Program

The American Heart Association and the National Cholesterol Education Program suggest you reduce fat calories and replace them with carbohydrate calories. But if you fail to lower total calories, which is also one of the options presented by these two agencies, you will not lose weight (barring exercise). This is precisely the scenario in which HDL usually will fall and small LDL and triglycerides usually will rise. A recent study by coauthor Dr. Mary Flynn confirms this. In a controlled diet study Flynn gave twenty people a diet that derived 37 percent of its calories from fat and measured their cholesterol and triglyceride levels. She then gave

Science, Consensus, and Self-Fulfilling Prophecies

We are all influenced by fads, beliefs, and myths, and top-rate research organizations are no exception. Husbanding scarce resources and looking to fund good research, they often, and quite understandably, adhere to the concensus opinion. Unfortunately, this sometimes means they fail to fund research that challenges convention in favor of research that supports it. The danger is that science becomes an exercise in making self-fullfilling prophecies.

In 1994 Mary Flynn, along with a cardiology colleague, confronted this problem when they wrote a research proposal to examine the effects of a diet rich in monounsaturated fats compared with an American Heart Association diet. Given the observed benefit of similar diets in Crete and southern Italy, one would think there would be a strong interest in studying these diets. Wrong. Here is what the reviewer of the proposal wrote:

> This is a well-designed study which should be able to answer the questions posed. The only observation is that the research question itself may be of limited interest. The merging consensus about dietary recommendations for maximal health seems to be to reduce total fat intake.

Translation: We have already decided that the way to go is a low-fat diet for all Americans, so we are not interested in finding out whether a diet of well-selected fats might be better than a low-fat diet. This reviewer—and he was typical—was so devoted to the consensus that he would not fund research that challenged it. Pretty soon most researchers get the message: In order to fund their work and pay their mortgages, they had better start submitting projects that conform to the party line, or start driving a cab.

the same group a diet that contained 25 percent of calories from fat but kept the total number of calories precisely the same by increasing carbohydrates. The low-fat diet was essentially the diet recommended by the National Cholesterol Education Program. She found that the low-fat diet lowered levels of HDL cholesterol, raised triglyceride levels, and basically left the levels of bad LDL cholesterol unchanged. Hardly optimal.

If you go on a low-fat diet and *do* lose weight or exercise, you may avoid elevated triglyceride levels. But usually this is not the case. Millions of Americans are eating low-fat, high-carbohydrate food and failing to lose weight. In fact, they're gaining weight. As they do their triglyceride levels climb, their HDL levels fall, and many will develop smaller, more aggressive LDL that is highly prone to oxidize and cause heart disease.

The Mediterranean Diet and Triglycerides

One of the great advantages of the Mediterranean diet is that it offers the possibility of optimizing your lipid profile with the judicious use of olive oil. By replacing some carbohydrate calories with olive oil calories, you can lower your triglyceride levels and maintain or even raise your HDL levels even before you lose a pound. On this kind of diet, you will be less likely to develop carbohydrate-induced small LDL. If you reduce total calories, you will lose weight, and your lipids will improve further.

Consider the case of Tom Tasca. In 1988 Tom was concerned about a cholesterol level of 209. He also had a reasonable triglyceride level of 128. His greatest concern at the time should have been his low HDL level of 34. However, he and his doctor were most focused on his total cholesterol, and so he went on a low-fat diet. On the kind of low-fat diet advocated by the National Cholesterol Education Program, his total cholesterol dropped to 175, but his triglyceride level shot up to 234, and his HDL level plummeted to a dangerous 26. Next he tried niacin, but developed severe itching and had to stop. Finally, he came to Dr. Mary Flynn, and she put him on a diet lower in calories but higher in fat, primarily olive oil. He dropped weight, and, as one would have predicted, his lipids improved dramatically. His total cholesterol came down to 171, his triglyceride level plunged to an outstanding 69, and his HDL level shot up to a very respectable 43.

Low-fat fanaticism has made this kind of olive oil–based diet verboten to Americans, and they are suffering the consequences. Not only have low-fat diets often failed to control their weight, for many they also will have a deleterious effect on triglyceride and HDL levels while promoting small LDL. Yes, a low-fat diet is better than always eating at McDonalds, and cutting out saturated fat is a good thing. But the categorical condemnation of all fat is unwarranted and dangerous to your health. It makes much more sense to recommend a broader spectrum of diets and at least to include one of the healthiest diets in the world—the olive oil–based Mediterranean diet.

7 Low-Fat Diets and the Silent Killer

In the 1980s an internationally renowned insulin and lipid researcher named Dr. Gerald Reaven described a deadly syndrome to which he gave the ominous name syndrome X. This syndrome as he originally described it consisted of four principal characteristics: central obesity, hypertension, lipid abnormalities—especially low HDL and high triglycerides—and insulin resistance. Realizing that low-fat diets had the potential to worsen syndrome X, Reaven was one of the early solitary voices warning against national policies advocating that all Americans pursue low-fat diets. His warnings have mostly gone unheeded. Since then, with the benefit of further research—especially on the dangers of small LDL—others have refined the syndrome and given it other, usually less dramatic names such as the metabolic syndrome. This later term, coined by another internationally famous nutrition researcher, Dr. Scott Grundy, has expanded the syndrome to include seven characteristics. Not surprisingly, he too has warned against the blanket banning of fat and the nearly universal prescription of low-fat diets. Whatever you call it, syndrome X or the metabolic syndrome, it is deadly—and with our current obesity epidemic, it is common. It is probably what killed the man whose resuscitation we described in Chapter 1. What makes it even more deadly is that most people afflicted with this syndrome aren't even aware they have it. It is a silent killer. The metabolic syndrome—son of syndrome X—includes the following seven characteristics:

1. Central Obesity. People who carry fat around their waists are at a higher risk of death than people who carry fat elsewhere.

2. Hypertension. Obesity puts people at risk for hypertension, a common feature of the metabolic syndrome. Even if the hypertension is mild, as it often is, combined with the other features of the metabolic syndrome it results in significantly increased risk.

3. High Triglycerides. The triglyceride elevation in this syndrome is, by today's official standards, often mild—certainly not the level that would get most doctors excited. Worse yet, doctors often elevate fasting triglyceride levels, so they put people with elevated triglyceride levels on low-fat diets. If their patients fail to lose a significant amount of weight, which often happens, that not only worsens their triglyceride levels, it also exacerbates the whole metabolic syndrome.

4. Low HDL. Low HDL and high triglyceride levels go hand in hand. However, the low HDL levels associated with the metabolic syndrome are often mild and frequently go unrecognized by

Low-Fat Diet Warning Label

The metabolic syndrome occurs when abnormal blood lipids, insulin, hypercoagulability, hypertension, and obesity all come together as dangerous conspirators. Low-fat diets without weight loss or exercise can become coconspirators. Low-fat diets should come with a warning: *You are being put on this diet to lower your risk of heart disease by lowering your LDL cholesterol levels. However, you also run the risk of increasing your levels of triglycerides and small LDL, and decreasing your levels of HDL. To prevent this from happening and to maximize the benefit of this diet, you must decrease the number of calories you consume and lose weight. Weight loss will prevent your triglyceride levels from rising. You should also exercise, because it has been shown that exercise can prevent your triglyceride levels from rising and your HDL levels from falling when you are on a low-fat, high-carbohydrate diet.*

That's a rather long-winded warning, but that's what people need to be told. Yet I have never heard a physician, a dietitian, Dr. Dean Ornish, or the National Cholesterol Education Program issue this warning with the low-fat diets they advocate. But the data are quite clear: low-fat, high-carbohydrate diets often raise triglyceride levels and lower HDL levels in the absence of weight loss and exercise.

physicians. Worse, our research showed that 82 percent of physicians surveyed didn't know that low-fat diets lower HDL levels, so they frequently put patients on low-fat, high-carbohydrate diets that lower HDL levels even more.

5. Small LDL. Along with elevated triglyceride and low HDL levels, small LDL is a common feature of the metabolic syndrome. Once again we see that low-fat diets may contribute to the metabolic syndrome by causing many people to shift from large LDL to small LDL, which is more likely to become oxidized.

6. Tendency of Blood to Clot. For reasons that are not completely clear, people who are afflicted with many of the conditions listed here also suffer from a predisposition of their blood to clot, called hypercoagulability. This is good if you cut yourself; it's bad if you are at risk for heart disease. Blood that clots too easily helps block up the coronary arteries and reduces blood flow to the heart. Recent research has suggested that the tendency to clot may be related in some way to low HDL. Scientists from Spain found that HDL provokes the production of prostacyclin, a hormone-like substance that inhibits blood clotting. The low HDL in the metabolic syndrome may therefore contribute to the tendency of blood to clot in this syndrome.

7. Insulin Resistance. One of the many functions of insulin is to attach to insulin receptors on cells so glucose can get into cells to be used for energy. When insulin or the insulin receptors aren't working properly and glucose has difficulty getting into hard-working cells like muscle cells, heart cells, and brain cells, the blood glucose level rises. We call that condition insulin resistance, and it can lead to diabetes. Diabetes damages blood vessels and puts people at risk for heart disease, blindness, kidney failure, and many other problems. Severe diabetics require insulin shots.

Insulin resistance is very closely associated with obesity because as people get more obese, the number of active insulin receptors on cells, the place where insulin attaches, goes down, and those remaining insulin receptors function less efficiently. As obesity increases, the body churns out more insulin to flog the remaining insulin receptors so that glucose can get into the cells.

Insulin resistance often goes unrecognized because we don't often check insulin levels in the blood. But insulin resistance and chronically elevated insulin levels can be deadly. Insulin resistance carries with it a dramatic increase in the risk of death from heart disease, and some maintain that it is at least as good a predictor of heart disease as cholesterol levels. Insulin resistance is intimately related to obesity and is strongly linked to all the other components of the metabolic syndrome.

The good news is that weight loss seems to promote the creation of new, more efficient insulin receptors. This in turn causes a reduction in insulin resistance, and insulin levels go down. The bad news is that starchy carbohydrates and sugar, which are often consumed in great quantities in low-fat, high carbohydrate diets, are among the most potent stimulators of insulin release. This causes even higher insulin levels in people whose insulin levels are already too high. Furthermore, low-fat diets that fail to promote weight loss may actually exacerbate insulin resistance and the metabolic syndrome.

> When we asked physicians to define a low-fat diet, 70 percent of those responding said a low-fat diet was less than 20 percent fat (far lower than the goal set by the American Heart Association). Yet 96 percent of these physicians did not know that a diet so low in fat would raise triglycerides.

Each of the elements of the metabolic syndrome, taken separately, increases the risk of heart disease and death. When added together, the risk of death skyrockets. And that's what makes this syndrome so dangerous. Each of the elements is related to all the others, and they tend to travel together.

The other thing that makes this syndrome so dangerous is that it is largely invisible. Other than having a big belly, many elements of this syndrome often go undetected. Certainly I've never heard EMTs radio the emergency room to say that they were bringing in a sixty-year-old man with "the metabolic syndrome in cardiac arrest." But much of the time that's exactly what they are doing. The man I described in the opening pages of this book probably had it. He's like millions of Americans walking around today with a host of mild abnormalities that go undetected but add up to a big risk. Hypertension is often mild and may not ring any alarm bells. The same is true for low HDL levels and elevated triglyceride levels. Insulin resistance and the tendency for blood to clot require tests that are often done only in the research setting. And so, though potentially deadly, these mild abnormalities often go unnoticed.

What's worse, if action is taken, it often comes in the form of a low-fat diet. As we know, most people on low-fat diets generally don't lose weight. As a result triglyceride and insulin levels may rise, HDL may fall even more, and in many people more LDL may shift to the smaller form. Although effects will vary from person to person depending on genetics, diet, and the degree of exercise and weight loss, low-fat diets may increase risk of heart disease for millions of Americans with the metabolic syndrome.

Between 1987 and 1994, deaths from heart disease went down, but the rate at which people developed heart disease went up. The reason for this good news/bad news dichotomy isn't exactly clear, but it is disturbing and invites speculation. It suggests to us that while fancy procedures and drugs have enabled us to save more people once they have their first heart attack or develop angina, we still have not succeeded in preventing the development of heart disease in the first place. This failure of prevention occurs in the face of a decrease in smoking and reduction in dietary fat. It is

Low-Fat Diets May Increase Coronary Artery Disease

In 1985 the Consensus Conference of the National Institute of Health issued a statement recommending that all Americans go on low-fat diets. Afterwards, Gerald Reaven renounced lipid research arguing that such blanket recommendations were ill advised because such diets may not be beneficial for all Americans, including many elderly and those with insulin resistance, as in syndrome X. He wrote, "there is reason to be believe that changes in plasma, insulin... triglyceride... and HDL... which might occur in response to low-fat/high-carbohydrate diets would actually increase the risk of CAD [coronary artery disease]". Time passing and further research seem only to have further validated his concern.

almost certain that sedentary behavior, the skyrocketing intake of sugar and other carbohydrates, increasing obesity, and an epidemic of the metabolic syndrome play a very important role in the increased incidence of heart disease. Weight loss is critical to reversing the metabolic syndrome. Although low-fat, high-carbohydrate diets are often meant to help people lose weight and keep it off, they often fail. As Dr. Scott Grundy has said, "There is a growing realization... that decreasing the percentage of total... fat is not the solution to worsening obesity in the United States...." And so low-fat diets, as commonly prescribed, may only be making matters worse.

8 Dean Ornish:
King of the Fat Phobes

Dr. Dean Ornish is probably the leading advocate for extremely low-fat or even no-fat diets. He has turned his fat phobia into a great career, writing best-selling books, lecturing, and appearing on TV. These days he even consults with food-industry behemoth ConAgra, so it can cash in on the low-fat/no-fat diet craze he helped create. Ornish practically forbids fat in every form—not just in meat and dairy, but in fish as well. He wants you to get your healthy omega-3 fatty acids from seaweed, soy, and purslane (an herb)—fat chance. Ornish doesn't want a drop of olive oil to touch your lips and also takes a very dim view of red wine. In short, the Mediterranean diet, one of the most heart-healthy diets in the world, is forbidden. This has been one of the most unfortunate consequences of the low-fat lie in general.

Ornish has been amazingly influential. The simplistic anti-fat message that Americans have been bombarded with—the message that makes them reach for the olestra-laden, trans fat–laced WOW

Doritos or try to live on plain steamed broccoli until they can't take it anymore—is the very message Ornish has been pushing.

Why is Dr. Ornish the King of the Fat Phobes? Unlike many diet gurus, Dean Ornish has done some serious, valuable, and original scientific research. He uses that research to back up his low-fat arguments.

So what's the problem? His original research can be valuable in guiding the treatment of heart patients in an intensive clinical setting, but it simply does not prove the claim he is really famous for, which is that Americans should cut virtually all fat from their diets.

Dean Ornish's Excellent Adventure

In 1990 Dr. Ornish and his colleagues published the results of a year-long experiment in *Lancet*, a British medical journal. The article, "Can Lifestyle Changes Reverse Coronary Heart Disease?", showed from a small, twenty-two–person study that heart-disease patients who followed a rigorous program that included a very-low-fat diet could dramatically reverse coronary artery disease. The arteries of the patients who followed the program opened up, and they also had fewer symptoms—less chest pain and fewer heart attacks—than those who did not.

A follow-up study published in 1998 tracked the progress of these patients over the next five years. Most of those who stayed with the regimen experienced further opening of their blood vessels, while most in the control group worsened. Ornish and his colleagues had demonstrated that lifestyle changes could reverse heart disease and that the improvements could be sustained over five years.

That's great. But the study did not provide evidence that Americans should cut all fat, including monounsaturated fat, out of

Vegetarians and Mediterraneans

In defending his diet, Dr. Ornish asserts that millions of people around the world are vegetarians. But as food critic Jeffrey Steingarten points out in his book *The Man Who Ate Everything*, only 6.7 percent of Americans claim to be vegetarians. And 40 percent of these "vegetarians" say they eat fish or poultry every week. In other words, they are eating more like Mediterraneans than vegetarians.

their diets. It did not even prove that the low-fat diet itself was the most important factor in reversing heart disease. Here's why.

First, the Ornish regimen, called the Lifestyle Heart Trial, did a lot more than put patients on a low-fat diet. They had to follow a complex, difficult regimen that dramatically transformed their lives—and they had an elaborate, expensive coaching and psychological support system to help them do it. The Ornish program included not just one lifestyle change—the extremely low-fat diet—but five, including exercise (lots of it), meditation (lots of it), group therapy (ditto), and weight loss (you guessed it, a lot).

Despite the breadth and intensity of these changes, Ornish focuses mostly on the role of his ultra-low-fat "Reversal Diet." He asserts that his no-fat diet "is the most effective diet for lowering cholesterol and preventing heart disease." Unfortunately his experiment doesn't prove his claim. This is an example of one of the most fundamental errors you can make in science. You remember: Your eighth-grade science teacher told you that in science you should "isolate your variables" and test one at a time. For example, if she told you to figure out which of two things turns water solid, adding green food coloring or putting it in a freezer, you would not add green food coloring to a glass of water and then put the same glass in the freezer. You would take two different glasses of water, freeze one and add food coloring to the other, and see which turned solid. If you did both at the same time you couldn't prove which intervention made the water solid. You could only draw the conclusion that it was *either* the green food coloring or the lower temperature, or both. Similarly, Ornish required five life changes at the same time; therefore, we don't know which interventions were more effective.

Ornish does not make exagerated claims in his scientific papers. When he is writing for scientists, he writes like a scientist. When writing for the public, however, he discusses the other lifestyle changes, but sends the message that it's cutting the fat that does the trick. For instance, when promoting his ultra-low-fat diet he says, "The comparison group of the Lifestyle Heart Study made moderate changes in diet yet felt worse." The message here is that it was the diet that made the difference.

But what about the stress management, exercise, weight loss, and group therapy? Ornish seems to play them down by frequently using the phrase "diet and other lifestyle changes," as if these changes were a chorus of less significant players. Maybe these changes were so obviously trivial that common sense tells us that cutting out the fat was the important part, just as we would know that it was the freezer, not the food coloring, that made the water solid. However, the other interventions *were* massive, sort of like a combination of a monastery and marine boot camp, and very relevant to treating heart disease. Here's what Ornish's patients had to do in addition to cutting out all fat and all meat— including fish:

Exercise. Each recruit had a customized exercise program based on the results of exercise stress tests. During the first year of the study they exercised, on average, one hour a day, five days a week. Five years later they were still exercising three and a half hours a week, usually spread over four sessions a week.

How much exercise is that? To put it in perspective, only about 4 percent of American men over age fifty-nine exercise three or more times a week, and the number who exercise five times or five hours a week is miniscule.

We know that exercise alone can have a dramatic impact on cardiac risk and can even reverse heart disease—even without dietary changes and weight loss. For instance, doctors from Heidelberg, Germany, did studies in which they put heart patients on a low-fat diet and encouraged them to exercise. They found that in the first year only those who exercised vigorously five or six times a week (like those in the Ornish group) reversed their heart disease. Those who exercised less worsened, even though they were on the same low-fat diet. In this study it was exercise, not diet, that made the crucial difference in reversing heart disease. Ornish doesn't emphasize these studies—but he should.

Exercise tends to raise HDL levels and lower triglyceride levels. However, despite vigorous exercise, the Ornish group showed an undesirable tendency toward lower HDL levels and higher triglyceride levels. It seems that the low-fat diet was just too much of a carbohydrate load to overcome, even with vigorous exercise.

Lose Weight. Ornish does not actually list this as one of his lifestyle changes, but he should. All of the patients on the Ornish regimen lost a significant amount of weight—an average of twenty-three and a half pounds in the first year. Even though the patients gained back an average of eleven pounds, five years later they were still thirteen and a half pounds lighter.

That's no surprise. In this study Ornish's low-fat diet is also a low-calorie diet, about 1,800 calories, and, as we know, when it comes to weight loss it's the calories that count. On average, an 1,800-calorie, monounsaturated fat–based diet would have produced the same weight loss in most people, especially with all that exercise.

Just as with exercise, we know that weight loss alone will make us more heart healthy: Weight loss alone seems to have independent beneficial effects on blood pressure, HDL and LDL cholesterol, triglycerides, and insulin regardless of whether one's diet is high fat or low fat. But in Ornish's study, HDL and triglyceride levels failed to improve despite weight loss.

Meditate. The recruits were also trained in various methods of relaxation, stress reduction, and meditation. During the first year they meditated an unbelievable ninety minutes a day. Even after five years, they were still meditating almost an hour a day.

Did the meditation matter? Very likely. Reducing stress and negative emotions has been shown to reduce cholesterol and symptoms of heart disease.

No-Fat Diet vs. Exercise vs. Weight Loss

Exercise, weight loss, and stress reduction: Each one is known to promote heart health, and all three probably help explain the dramatic improvement in Ornish's patients.

Ornish's diet is aimed at keeping fat consumption down to an astonishing 7 to 10 percent fat. Practically speaking, that makes it a no-fat diet, because the only way to go that low is to eliminate every gram of fat you can identify. A few grams will inevitably slip by, so if you want to meet the goal you must develop a fanatical, zero-tolerance, no-fat state of mind. Some of his patients became so fat-phobic they had to be prescribed a little flaxseed oil to lower the risk of any fat-based nutritional deficiencies.

The bottom line is that Ornish's study does not show that a no-fat diet alone will reverse heart disease. His study does not tell us anything about what would have happened to those patients without exercise, weight loss, or meditation. In fact, from what we know from the German studies, exercise seems to be a more important factor in reversing heart disease. Ornish's study has shown only that all the interventions taken together are effective, but not which ones helped, which ones hurt, and which ones made no difference.

Group Therapy, Too

But wait a minute. These patients stuck to their diets, stuck to their exercise, stuck to their meditation, and kept off most of their weight—for five years! How did they do it? We all know that the big problem with tough exercise regimens and draconian, tasteless diets is that people don't stick to them. But these folks did.

That takes us to Ornish's final lifestyle change, and it's a big one. Every participant received intensive psychological and emotional support to keep them on the program. Before they even began the study, recruits had to attend a week-long retreat in which they received highly concentrated instruction. After the study began, the recruits were required to meet twice a week for four hours to participate in professionally-led group-support meetings. While participants used these groups for mundane purposes such as exchanging recipes, they also used them to deal with issues of anger and communication. Ornish says that these groups took on the characteristics of a small community, reinforcing the group's goals.

In other words, over the course of five years each member of the group received the equivalent of as much as two thousand hours of group therapy and a great interpersonal support system, with powerful group values and moral reinforcement. Those group sessions, the dedication of Ornish and his patients to complete the study, and the powerful personal motives of the patients—all of whom had life-threatening heart disease—probably had a lot to do with why these twenty people were able to stay with the program.

So Ornish's approach worked fine for a small, intense, and expensive experiment with highly motivated people who were otherwise facing bypass surgery or death. But in the real world, who can live like that?

That may be why Ornish does not concisely spell out the details of his experimental regimen in his popular books. Sure, he waxes eloquent about lifestyle changes, especially the meditation—but he doesn't present them in their full paramilitary-monastic glory. He doesn't emphasize that to emulate his patients you would have to meditate ninety minutes a day, seven days a week; exercise religiously for five hours a week; go to marathon meetings twice a week; eat an 1,800-calorie, vegetarian, no-fat diet; and drop almost twenty-four pounds.

Of course he doesn't. Nobody would buy *that* book.

Dr. Ornish and Pop Science

When he writes for a popular audience, Dr. Ornish often selectively cites evidence, makes exaggerated claims, and sometimes

Dr. Ornish's Catch-22

Dr. Ornish pushes his 10 percent-fat Reversal Diet, which has recently acquired a trendier name—the Life Choice Diet— probably to complement the Life Choice Special Nutrition line of foods he helped ConAgra develop. But he briefly mentions a kinder, gentler diet—the Prevention Diet. Here he allows an occasional dose of canola oil or skinless chicken, but only on one very stringent condition: that your total cholesterol level stays below 150. Unfortunately, that excludes about 95 percent of U.S. adults. In fact, the twenty-two participants in the original Ornish Lifestyle Heart Trial couldn't get that low with all five lifestyle changes. Their average cholesterol level was 188 after five years. The catch-22 is that almost no one will qualify for the Prevention Diet, and those who do probably don't need it.

even tries to prove his points with studies that actually show something quite different.

In his books Ornish implies that his extremely low-fat diet is more effective than the American Heart Association Diet or olive oil–based diets like the Mediterranean diet. But his research supports neither claim. In fact there is no research, his or anyone else's, showing his model is superior to the Mediterranean model, and there are lots of reasons to think otherwise.

Ornish ignores the healthy Mediterranean diet data and proclaims, "Don't listen to what anyone tells you—olive oil is bad for you." In his book *Everyday Cooking with Dr. Dean Ornish* he specifically attacks olive oil and claims that "the more olive oil you eat, the higher your cholesterol will rise...." Unfortunately Ornish doesn't seem to know the scientific evidence. There is no evidence that shows that olive oil is bad for you, and the only cholesterol olive oil will raise is your good HDL cholesterol.

His book, with the unfortunate title *Eat More Weigh Less* (the last thing Americans need to be told is to eat more), sometimes misquotes or misinterprets the scientific research. For instance, on page twenty-five he argues for low-fat/high-carbohydrate diets by citing studies showing that these diets increase a certain type of thyroid hormone. He then goes on to explain this thyroid hormone increases metabolism, causing us to burn more calories and lose weight. Sounds good. Unfortunately, these scientific studies show something quite different from what Ornish claims. Yes, the Ornish-style diet did increase the levels of this thyroid hormone in all three studies. But the one study that actually measured metabolic rate showed that it went down on both diets but especially on the high-carbohydrate diet—just the opposite of what Ornish suggested. Furthermore, that same study showed the patients actually lost less weight on an Ornish-style diet and lost more weight on a high-fat/low-carbohydrate diet.

On page twenty-six Ornish states that insulin levels rise when you lose weight by eating less. That's not true. Insulin goes down when you lose weight by any means. Furthermore, low-fat, high-carbohydrate diets like his are notorious for raising insulin levels. That's why the American Diabetes Association has rightly avoided fat-phobic diets.

He then cites on page thirty-two a study by Chen Junshi, a researcher from China, and claims that the study shows that increased fat intake correlated with increased weight. Again in reality the study shows something different from what he suggests—dietary fat is not related to increased weight.

Different Strokes

If you can quit your job, attend marathon meetings, meditate daily, exercise religiously, and adhere to a highly restrictive, no-fat, vegetarian diet such as the one Ornish prescribes, then go ahead. But most Americans, even those facing life-threatening illness, will find it impossible to embrace the whole Ornish program, or even just the diet.

Studies have shown that even highly motivated people have a hard time eating less than 20 percent fat for long. What if you had to give up all fat *and* all meat at the same time, for a lifetime? No way.

That's why there probably will never be more than a few good men, or women, in the Holy Ornish Diet Corps. And that's why we think it's wrong to create the impression that this arduous regimen is the only way to health.

Not cut out for the Corps? Don't worry. The more simpatico Mediterranean diet offers an alternative you can live with—and probably better and longer. After all, what good is a diet if you won't eat it?

We could go on, but you get the idea. Ornish's popular books frequently have claims that he can't prove or are flat-out wrong. The bottom line is that while Ornish's no-fat diet may have reduced total cholesterol, it didn't produce the optimal lipid profile. It failed to raise HDL levels and lower triglyceride levels—despite weight loss and exercise. Ornish claims that a fall in HDL levels caused by diet is harmless, but much research suggests that higher HDL levels are much healthier. Adding a little olive oil would have raised HDL levels while lowering LDL and triglyceride levels—and provided a healthy dose of phytochemicals and antioxidants to boot. Had Ornish done this, as Dr. Frank Sachs, a Harvard researcher and former Ornish colleague, has written, "They [the patients] might have had even more improvement."

Ornish doesn't tell you about it, but there is much evidence to suggest that a Mediterranean-style, monounsaturated fat–based diet that tastes good, ensures carotene absorption, raises HDL levels, and lowers triglyceride and LDL levels would more effectively treat heart disease. The Lyon Heart study in France showed a dramatic reduction in heart disease symptoms—reductions comparable to Ornish's group—when patients were put on a Mediterranean diet. Even more impressive, five years later the Mediterranean diet group enjoyed a 61 percent lower risk of cancer and a 56 percent lower rate of death compared with a control group. And this was in three hundred patients, not just twenty-two.

> Results of the Nurses' Health Study reveal that women who ate more than five ounces of nuts a week had one-third fewer heart attacks than those who never ate nuts. Unfortunately, no nuts for Dr. Ornish's patients because they contain fat.

Ornish claims that his diet "is the world's healthiest diet for most adults." But in light of this study, he still has a lot to prove. Furthermore, the Lyon Heart study did not require additional exercise, meditation, or group therapy, so we can say that it was the Mediterranean diet—the diet alone—that made the difference.

Dining Out with Dr. Dean

Dr. Ornish writes a lot about loneliness in his books. Now we know why—no one would want to eat with him. This is the experience of *New York Times* reporter Gina Kolata, who went to dinner with Ornish:

> One evening last spring, Dr. Ornish started with Caesar salad, which he ordered with dressing on the side. When the salad came, he ignored the dressing, along with the Parmesan cheese and croutons that were sprinkled over the lettuce. Dr. Ornish's "Caesar salad" was simply a handful of leaves of Romaine. His main course was a plate of steamed vegetables surrounding a scoop of plain white rice. No butter. No oil. Not even any spices. He drank water. No dessert. No coffee.

Not only will eating like this scare away your friends, it is not good for your health. There's a good chance Dr. Ornish didn't absorb many of the carotenoids in his oil-free salad and vegetables.

9 The High-Fat Fraud

Confronted with the hunger, frustration, and ultimately the failure of low-fat diets, millions of desperate Americans have turned to high-fat, high-protein diets. Only too willing to greet them are the peddlers of the high-fat fraud. Instead of casting fat as the villain, they claim fat is the savior and carbohydrates are the villain. Instead of being fat phobes, they are carb phobes. But their theories are just as flawed, and some of the advice they give can be downright dangerous. What's worse, they've got everyone—physician and layman alike—confused. And there is nothing more paralyzing than confusion. We'd like to clear things up.

Carb Phobes

Perhaps the earliest high-fat fraud book to be peddled in America was penned by a Romanian-born gynecologist, Dr. Herman Taller, in 1961. The title of this book, *Calories Don't Count,* has become a mantra for many on both sides of the great diet debate—both fat phobes and carb phobes. After all, nobody wants to count calories. Most of us can't even balance our checkbooks, never mind figure out the arithmetic total of calories we consume every day. That book has since been followed by the ultimate carb-phobic regimen—*Dr. Atkins's Diet Revolution* and *Dr. Atkins's New Diet Revolution.* (Old diet revolutionaries never die, they just get richer. Man the barricades! And let them eat steak, or whatever will keep them buying the book.) After that came *The Zone* by Barry Sears, Ph.D. The Zone diet is a sort of kinder, gentler Atkins diet with a heavier patina of science and New Age marketing. Another is the Sugar Busters diet, which was authored by a curious foursome from New Orleans. One is a French businessman who felt that a French- style, high-fat diet was just what Americans needed if they wanted to look like svelte Parisians. The other three are physicians from three different subspecialties—an endocrinologist, a gastroenterologist, and a cardiovascular surgeon. These guys aren't fly-by-night diet doctors; they are real physicians with good academic credentials who take care of real patients. They are all affiliated with university teaching hospitals. *Sugar Busters*, as the name suggests, focuses on sugar, a simple carbohydrate, but it also advises readers to avoid starchy carbohydrates.

Despite the different spin employed by these books, they are all based on the same biochemical theory that is the essence of the high-fat fraud: People gain weight because of insulin, not calories. They claim carbohydrates are bad because they stimulate insulin release. Indeed *The Zone* refers to a hormonal "Zone" in which insulin levels are minimized. At some point all these books claim that calories don't matter. You can eat all the protein and fat calories you want; as long as you don't eat insulin-stimulating carbohydrates, you won't store any calories, and you will lose weight.

Insulin—The Body's Gatekeeper

Insulin is a hormone with many complicated effects. Its most well-known function is its ability to control glucose—that is, the sugar level in the blood. When we eat, food is absorbed from our intestines. Carbohydrates are broken down into their simplest form—sugar—and end up in the blood, causing glucose levels to rise. Insulin is then released by the pancreas, bringing glucose levels back down to normal. How much and how quickly insulin is released depends in large part on how much and how quickly glucose enters the bloodstream.

Where does the sugar go when insulin lowers it? It goes into the cells—muscle cells, brain cells, heart cells, and other hard-working cells—to be used for energy. Insulin is like the gatekeeper of our cells. Without insulin, glucose can't get in, and our cells don't get nourished. The cells soon start looking for something else to eat, and that something is fat. Whenever insulin is not present, the body doesn't use fats normally, and ketones, the products of abnormal fat metabolism, are produced.

But insulin not only lets sugar in, it helps fat get in fat cells too. As we discussed earlier, insulin influences an enzyme called lipoprotein lipase (LPL), which enables fat to enter muscle cells for energy use and into fat cells for storage. If insulin is the gatekeeper, LPL is the gatekeeper's key. When insulin levels are high, LPL at the muscle is suppressed while LPL at the fat cell is stimulated. So elevated insulin, by its effect on LPL, facilitates entry of fat into the fat cell. On the other hand, when insulin is very low, fat doesn't enter the fat cell as easily.

According to the Sugar Busters version of the carb-phobe theory, if you avoid foods that stimulate insulin (i.e., carbohydrates), insulin levels will stay low, LPL at the fat cell will be inactive, and the door to the fat cell will close. With the door to the fat cell closed you won't be able to store any fat and you won't get fat. In other words, if you eat only nutrients that don't stimulate insulin (i.e., fat and protein), you won't get fat. That's why the authors claim it doesn't matter how many calories you eat—as long as none of them are from carbohydrates, you won't gain weight.

Would You Care for Some Ketones with Your Steak?

Dr. Robert Atkins peddles one of the most extreme versions of the high-fat fraud. He virtually forbids the consumption of all sugar and starch—especially for the first two weeks. He tries to shut insulin production down completely in order to create a condition called ketosis. Ketones are the abnormal metabolic products of fats, and they are produced when an insulin-deprived body uses fats for energy. When many ketones are produced, we say the body is in ketosis. Because ketones are acidic, they can cause the blood to become acidic. If the blood becomes extremely acidic, enzymes and organs don't function, and death ensues if the process is not reversed. This profound, life-threatening form of ketosis most often occurs when severe diabetics who produce no insulin are in extreme crisis. Even though these diabetics are eating and have a lot of sugar in their blood, they lack insulin and can't get the sugar into their cells. The starving cells scream for nourishment, and the body starts breaking down fat, but in the absence of insulin the cells can't use fat properly. Ketones are produced at an enormous rate, and these patients quickly spiral downward toward coma and death unless they receive insulin, fluids, and proper electrolytes.

But milder and less catastrophic forms of ketosis occur as well. When people starve and metabolize body fat to survive, they develop mild to moderate ketosis. People with lots of fat can exist in that state for months. By excluding almost all complex carbohydrates, Atkins tries to induce a ketotic state that is analogous to starvation. He claims this will cause two desirable effects. First, without insulin your cells can't get glucose, and your body breaks down its own fat stores for energy, causing you to lose weight. Second, he boasts that you can have all the eggs Benedict and steak you want without any regard for total calories, and you will lose weight without getting hungry.

But where do all the calories from the eggs Benedict go? I ran the Atkins, Zone, and Sugar Busters theories past Dr. Ralph DeFronzo, a former teacher of mine and one of the world's leading authorities on insulin. Always direct, DeFronzo said, "It's a lot of garbage. Where do you think these calories go? You don't excrete them. The answer is, you store them. If you lose weight it's because you're taking in fewer calories or burning more."

Dr. Atkins's Un-Revolutionary Low-Calorie Diet

People who lose weight on the Atkins diet do so because they are eating fewer calories. You might think it is impossible that people would consume fewer calories on this high-fat diet, but it isn't. Carbohydrates account for almost 50 percent of the calories in an average person's diet. If you suddenly eliminate 50 percent of your calories it would be difficult to compensate for that loss. We added up a daily total calorie count from a typical breakfast, lunch, and supper recommended by Atkins and it came to 1,400 to 1,500 calories, if you can actually eat that much fat and protein. Most obese women will lose weight on 1,500 calories a day, and most men will lose weight on 2,000 calories a day. Add to this calorie reduction the water weight you initially lose when you deplete the body of stored glucose (glycogen), and bingo—weight loss.

I actually tried this diet myself and found it difficult to find enough things to eat. After two weeks I was so sick of eating eggs, meat, and cheese three or four times a day that I couldn't take it anymore. I simply found it hard to eat that much fat and meat in the course of a day. I also found my mind was fuzzy, I was irritable, and I was spending a lot of time in the bathroom. After I almost passed out in the gym I had to stop working out. I lost about four pounds, but it probably had nothing to do with insulin or ketones. I lost the weight because I was consuming only about 1,800 calories a day on Atkins's low-calorie diet plan. True, I wasn't hungry. But it was clear my body didn't like being in ketosis. Finally, after two weeks, I had a plate of pasta, and the world looked right again.

Of course, that's just one man's experience. The question is, what does the research show? Guess what? There's practically none. Sure, Atkins, like Sears and the authors of *Sugar Busters*, cites all kinds of studies. But most of these "studies" are window dressing that fail to test the hypothesis. Both Atkins and Sears do come up with one controlled study to "prove" their carb-phobe hypotheses—a seriously flawed study that was published more than forty years ago in *Lancet*, a British medical journal. This study purported to show that in a group of patients on the same 1,000-calorie diet, those getting almost all their calories from fat or protein lost more weight than those getting almost all their calories from carbohydrates. But this study, conducted in an English hospital ward, was so poorly controlled that the authors even stooped to criticize their patients. They wrote, "Many of these patients had inadequate personalities. At worst they would cheat and lie, obtaining food from visitors, from trolleys touring the wards, and from neighboring patients." It's not hard to believe that patients on a 1,000-calorie carbohydrate diet were so hungry that they were driven to a life of crime. Those extra purloined calories could easily account for their failure to lose weight, and in fact similar studies several years later failed to show the same results. Although I would hardly call this irrefutable scientific proof, it is apparently good enough for these peddlers of the high-fat fraud.

Everybody Must Get Zoned

The Zone diet doesn't eliminate carbohydrates; it just cuts them down to 40 percent of total calories, while protein is pumped up to 30 percent and fats are held at 30 percent to create a ratio of 40:30:30 (carbohydrates: proteins: fats, respectively). Barry Sears also insists that you severely limit starchy carbohydrates like potatoes, pasta, and bread, which have a high glycemic index. The glycemic index, a scale developed by Dr. David Jenkins of the University of Toronto, ranks foods according to how likely they are to cause a surge of insulin-provoking glucose in the blood. Sears says that if you maintain this magical ratio of 40:30:30 you will be in the Zone and your body will work with the efficiency of a finely tuned carburetor. In this magical Zone you can eat to your heart's content because calories are irrelevant. All that matters is insulin, and with this food ratio insulin levels, and hence fat storage, are minimized. So powerful is the almighty Zone that, according to Sears, you will be able to "reset your genetic code" and "burn more fat watching TV than by exercising." But our genetic code is established at the moment of conception and, short of a radiation blast or some other DNA-damaging carcinogen, does not change. As for burning more fat while watching TV—please.

Like Atkins and the authors of *Sugar Busters*, Sears makes a great deal of the fact that where you find obesity you find high insulin levels. This leads him and the others to the conclusion that insulin causes obesity, and if you lower insulin levels you will magically get thin. Unfortunately, they've got it backward. As previously mentioned, elevated insulin levels are a sign of insulin resistance and are a consequence, not a cause, of obesity. As we put on weight, the body's insulin apparatus functions less efficiently, and it takes more and more insulin to accomplish the same task. Thus obesity causes insulin levels to go up; elevated insulin levels do not cause obesity. Sears's error is probably why Dr. Gerald Reaven, an internationally renowned expert on insulin, has been quoted by *New Yorker* science writer Malcolm Gladwell as saying, "I think he's full of it."

On the other hand, if you follow the Zone menu as prescribed by marketing wizard Barry Sears, you will probably lose weight, but not because you are in the all-powerful Zone. Sears has wrapped his scheme in the grandiose and complicated trappings of scientific terminology to disguise what is actually a quite mundane low-calorie diet. If you take a good look at the daily meal plans, they hover around 1,000 to 1,200 calories a day for women and 1,500 to 1,700 calories a day for men. That's the reason it works; it has nothing to do with the Zone.

Busting Up the Sugar Busters

After reading *Sugar Busters*, I had the feeling the authors are likable, very sincere fellows who really felt they were onto something revolutionary. Unfortunately, it doesn't make them right. Like Barry Sears, they make much of the capacity of high-glycemic foods, like potatoes and pasta, to stimulate insulin release. However, they fail to adequately emphasize that these foods are rarely eaten in isolation and that mixing starchy foods with a little fat dramatically lowers their glycemic index and their capacity to stimulate insulin release.

The authors also go into great detail about how insulin stimulates lipoprotein lipase to let fat into fat cells and theorize that if you promote insulin by eating sugar and starchy carbohydrates, you will store more fat. As we have seen before, weaving theories on the basis of single biochemical reactions is fraught with error. They conveniently ignore the biochemical "factoid" that Dean Ornish emphasizes: It takes less energy to store fat than carbohydrates. Who's right? Only an experiment can sort that out, and the authors of *Sugar Busters* haven't done one.

The authors of *Sugar Busters* see sugar as toxic and the root of all evil. While we certainly agree that Americans are drowning themselves in sugar and that it is responsible for much of the weight gain Americans have experienced over the past thirty years, a little sugar in your coffee won't kill you. Weight gain, if it occurs, comes not from the insulin sugar stimulates but from the calories it adds. You can eat a little sugar and lose weight as long as you reduce the total number of calories you consume. Researchers at Duke University put one group of people on a high-sugar but low-calorie diet and another group on a low-sugar diet with the same number of calories as the first group. According to Sugar Busters theory, those in the low-sugar group should have lost more weight. They didn't.

People probably lose weight on the Sugar Busters diet for the same reasons they may lose weight on the Zone or Atkins diet. By cutting way down on sugar and other carbohydrates, the diet eliminates calories wholesale. By pushing fat and protein, the diet promotes satiety. It has nothing to do with fancy insulin theories—it's simply a low-calorie diet.

The Burden of Proof

Given the "revolutionary" nature of these books and the nutritional theories they promote, you would think the authors would have tested their theories before selling them to the public.

They carry that burden of proof. Nothing fancy is required—just a small randomized trial to see if the insulin-based, calories-don't-count, carb-phobe hypothesis is right. Our recommendation for each would have been to get forty subjects and put half on a low-carbohydrate, high-fat diet and the other half on a high-carbohydrate, low-fat diet for at least six weeks and track the weight loss. Both groups would get the same number of calories. If these authors' theories are right—that calories don't count but insulin secretion does—those on the low-carbohydrate, high-fat diet should lose more weight. This isn't a hard study to do. All you need are forty people and a scale. But even though they have sold millions of books and made many millions of dollars, these authors haven't done the one simple thing they need to do to prove their theory. Makes you wonder.

> In our survey, 65 percent of physicians said they did not have enough nutrition knowledge to provide dietary advice to patients with lipid disorders.

Looking for a Few Good Studies

Because the authors didn't test their theories, we scoured the medical literature to see whether other researchers did. At first all we found were plenty of studies showing that people gain weight when you increase calories regardless of whether those calories come from fats or carbohydrates. Finally we turned up a study done by Dr. Mary Alice Kerns to test the Zone diet.

Kerns did exactly what Barry Sears and all these authors should have done before disregarding years of research and touting the efficacy of their new "revolutionary" theories. Kerns put one group of patients on a low-fat, high-carbohydrate diet and another group on a Zone-type diet. In both cases she kept the amount of calories precisely the same. What she found won't please Sears. She found that both groups lost the same amount of weight. Calories do appear to matter. In fact, in this study it was the only thing that mattered. After all of Sears's imaginative theorizing about losing more weight when you are in the Zone, Kerns found it didn't make an iota of difference. The truth is that if someone loses weight on the Zone diet it's not because of its effect on insulin, but probably because it is a low-calorie diet, albeit a complicated one. Barry Sears has basically tricked people into eating just another type of low-calorie diet and made a fortune doing it. And that's the high-fat fraud.

Kerns *did* find that the group who ate fewer carbohydrates and more fat had a better blood lipid profile. Both groups had a drop in cholesterol but the low carbohydrate group had better triglyceride and HDL levels. Though Dean Ornish and other fat phobes may find this final point hard to swallow, it's not surprising to us. We have said from the beginning that too many carbs can lower HDL and raise triglycerides. But unlike Atkins, Sears, and the *Sugar Busters* authors, we think the best way to prevent that is not to give up protein or saturated fat but to swap some carb calories for olive oil.

It was even harder to find a good study that looked at an Atkins-like diet. That's probably because there are few physicians and nutritionists willing to put their patients on a high-fat diet that induces ketosis. There is one exception, however, and that is the ketogenic diet to control seizures in children. For reasons that are not well understood, ketones, the products of fat metabolism, suppress seizures in children. So children who have seizures that can't be controlled with drugs are sometimes put on a ketogenic diet that is about 80 percent fat. If Atkins's theory is correct, these children should lose weight when they go on this diet, and increasing their caloric intake should not put the weight back on, because, according to Atkins, calories don't count.

I spoke to a few experts on the ketogenic diet at Johns Hopkins University, where the diet was developed, and elsewhere. Dr. John Freeman, a neurologist at Johns Hopkins, and his nutritionist both said that their experience didn't support the Atkins hypothesis. They found that these children, who were in a constant state of ketosis, gained and lost weight precisely as one would predict based on their caloric intake. If kids ate less because they found the diet unpleasant, they lost weight. If they were fed more calories, they gained the predicted amount of weight. Though this confirmed our impressions, including how difficult it was to stay on this diet for the long term, we still wanted to find a formal study of the issue.

Dr. Arthur Agatston, a cardiologist at the Mt. Sinai Medical Center in Miami, was being besieged by questions from his patients about high-fat, high-protein diets. He hadn't seen any good studies testing these diets, so he decided to do his own. He recruited seventy-eight patients and put them on an Atkins-like diet. He started them on a whopping 62 percent of calories from fat, 28 percent of calories from protein, and only 10 percent of calories from carbohydrates. He found that 77 percent of his patients lost weight, with 22 percent losing fifteen pounds or more. At first it seemed like Dr. Atkins, the embattled diet revolutionary, might be vindicated. So I asked Agatston the crucial question; How many calories did he allow on this diet? "We put no limitation on how many calories they could eat," he said. I was getting ready to eat crow, in unlimited quantities, myself. Then he added, "But people only ended up eating about 1,200 to 1,500 calories a day. They just got filled up on the fat and couldn't eat any more." This, of course, supports what we've been saying all along. First, fat is filling. Second, it's not fat, or carbohydrates, or insulin, or ketones that are most crucial to weight gain—it's calories that count. Atkins, like Sears and the authors of *Sugar Busters*, has fooled millions of people into eating a low-calorie diet— while he makes some high-calorie bucks.

It is extraordinary that even though these high-fat, high-protein, carb-phobe diets have been around, in one form or another, for almost forty years and have been used by millions of people, we could find only two studies that set out to formally examine them. This is what we have to go on, and at this time all the available evidence suggests that any diet that denies the importance of calories is fraudulent.

The Danger of Saturated Fat

But so what, you say. It doesn't matter why these diets work as long as I lose weight on them.

Well it matters a great deal. The Atkins diet recommends consuming saturated fat without restraint, and, as we know, saturated fat has been shown to raise levels of LDL cholesterol, which is strongly associated with heart disease. Atkins claims his diet is safe, and to prove the safety of saturated fats he cites all sorts of stories about folks whose cholesterol went down on his diet. No studies, just stories.

Let's accept his word that the stories are true. At first it may seem paradoxical that cholesterol would go down on a diet drenched in saturated fat. But not necessarily. Any diet that reduces calories through the gimmick of forbidding an entire category of food and thereby inducing weight loss generally causes a reduction in blood cholesterol. Weight loss causes blood cholesterol to drop. It would be far better to be on a diet that improved your cholesterol independently of weight loss and then protected that cholesterol from oxidation. A diet that didn't forbid whole categories of food but embraced food in a balanced and sensible way. A diet tested by time in the real world and one you could live with for a lifetime: the Mediterranean diet.

The Problem with Protein

We also think it's risky, over the long term, to consume the excessive amounts of protein recommended by the Zone, Atkins, and Sugar Busters diets. First, protein can leach calcium out of your system, and with osteoporosis already reaching epidemic proportions, we don't need diets that increase its risk. Second, excessive meat consumption is associated with heart disease and cancer. While some have tried to pin the blame for this entirely on saturated fat, there is evidence to suggest that for cancer at least, the problem is not the fat but carcinogens such as heterocyclic amines that are often found in seared meat. The association between meat consumption and colon cancer is very strong, and recent evidence has convincingly linked well-cooked meat to breast cancer. But it's not just the carcinogens; meat also has a substitution effect. By focusing excessively on meat, people fail to eat as many plant-based foods rich in antioxidants, phytochemicals, and fiber that can prevent cancer and heart disease. Finally, there is even some evidence that protein can bind to certain disease-fighting phytochemicals and inhibit their absorption. While absolute vegetarianism is an impractical and unnecessary objective for most people, meat should be minimized.

Oh, well, you point out, protein doesn't have to come from meat—you can get it from other sources like beans and tofu. True. And if you get protein from those sources, great. But I guarantee you that if you encourage Americans to eat a diet that is 30 percent protein, they won't be getting it from beans and tofu. They'll get it from Big Macs and porterhouse steaks.

Calories Do Count

In the end we may discover that certain people, in subtle biochemical ways, may be more sensitive to certain kinds of macronutrients like fat or carbohydrates. But the evidence suggests that in the real world these differences are inconsequential when it comes to weight gain and weight loss. It's calories—how many you consume and how many you burn—that count. While some people with a thrifty body chemistry may store calories easily and others may burn them quickly because of their faster metabolism, the coin of the realm is still calories. So the answer is not weird diets that forbid pasta, bread, and potatoes. The answer is a lifelong way of eating that fills you up on relatively few calories, coupled with a daily brisk walk. If you do this, you will lose weight. Period. You may not look like Christie Brinkley or Brad Pitt, but you will look and feel much better than you do today.

You should be suspicious of any diet that advocates disregarding calories and eating as much as you want. While it is true that you can use fat in a way that helps you consume fewer calories, there is no biochemical hocus-pocus involved. It's just that fat fills you up. This is something the Mediterraneans have known for thousands of years and seems novel only because we have spent the past forty years trying to deny the truth and time-tested wisdom of this simple, commonsense observation. But it is critical to choose the right fat, and the best fat to choose is olive oil. So however well-meaning Atkins, Sears, and the foursome from New Orleans may be, stay away from a steady diet of saturated fats— steak, hamburgers, butter, and eggs Benedict. Although it won't kill you to have some saturated fat every now and then, over a lifetime a steady dose will. Telling you differently is a high-fat fraud.

10 Eat Fast Food, Die Younger, Leave an Obese Corpse

W hen **James Dean** said, "Live fast, die young, leave a beautiful corpse" in the 1950s, Americans were much thinner, and fast food was a new invention. Today Americans are simply too chubby to live as fast as the lean 1950s idol. Instead they eat fast food, die younger than they should, and leave increasingly obese corpses. Along with smoking, substance abuse, and inactivity, fast food presents one of the greatest public health threats to Americans today. Fast food is almost universally dangerous and should probably carry a warning from the surgeon general. It contains meat-based carcinogens, is high in total calories and saturated fat, and is a principal source of trans fat.

Americans are always looking to shave a few seconds off everything—even eating. Fast food is a $103 billion industry, and more than 25,000 new fast-food restaurants opened between 1996 and 1998. In a country obsessed with immediate gratification and conspicuous consumption, what could be more seductive than the capacity to consume excessively at a moment's notice? The dominance of the fast-food culture makes it possible to have almost continual, unhealthy, moveable feasts—daily.

Not only is the food dangerous, but it promotes a lifestyle and culture that are also dangerous. Our lives are fast, frenetic, and commercial. Food should be our sanctuary from the madness, not part of it. It's no accident that Dave Thomas, the happy CEO of Wendy's who pushes the company's burgers on TV, had a coronary bypass operation several years ago. As we can see on more recent commercials, he's dropped a few pounds, but that hasn't stopped him from hawking his products to the rest of us.

Fast Food and Fat Kids

American children are not eating well. Approximately 30 percent of American children are obese, up more than 50 percent in the past twenty years. In general, American children eat too much, and much of what they eat is unhealthy. A study sponsored by the National Research Council and the Institute of Medicine revealed that despite poverty and poorer access to health care, immigrant children were actually healthier than their American-born counterparts, having fewer short- and long-term health problems. The researchers noted that immigrant children ate fewer processed foods and more fruits, grains, and vegetables. Unfortunately, as time goes on, the immigrant children acquire the unhealthy eating habits of American-born children. As Rubin Rumbaut, one of the researchers cited in the report, says, "The McDonaldization of the world is not necessarily progress when it comes to nutritious diets."

The Killer Clown

We are surrounded by trans fats in many of the foods we eat, but the single largest dose we are likely to get is still the seemingly innocuous, cholesterol-free french fries from Wendy's, Burger King, or McDonalds. McDonalds is the largest source of these potentially fatal fries.

McDonalds understands that food is a cultural issue, and it spends more than a half a billion dollars a year promoting the McDonalds culture of eating. That culture is even penetrating public schools, places where children should be learning to make healthy lifestyle choices. Fast-food chains are now contracting with public schools to provide unhealthy, trans fat–laden lunches for our children.

In an effort to attract children to the McDonalds culture of eating, the company has created a cultural icon that rivals some of the most universally recognized symbols in Western culture. According to *Rolling Stone* magazine, 96 percent of school children surveyed could recognize Ronald McDonald, making him second only to Santa Claus in name recognition, and the Golden Arches are more recognized than the Christian cross. Every day Ronald McDonald, the killer clown, seduces more and more children to eat fast foods that may cause them to become obese and to live shorter lives. Ronald McDonald is just as dangerous as Joe Camel.

Fast Food and Trans Fats

Most people know that fast food is not good for you, but many don't realize how dangerous it really is. They probably know about the calories, saturated fat, and maybe even the potential carcinogens in the beef. And they may even know about the dangers of ingesting *E. coli* bacteria from ground beef. But maybe they think they can escape the worst of it by skipping the burger and having the Chicken McNuggets or the french fries. After all, fries are just potatoes cooked in vegetable oil, right? Unfortunately the fries may be worse than the burger. Why? Trans fats.

Trans fats are man-made fats that were virtually unknown to humans until 1911, when Procter & Gamble, the people who brought you olestra, first marketed Crisco. Before Crisco, if you wanted to make a pie crust you needed to use lard or beef tallow as your solid fat source. But Procter & Gamble discovered that adding hydrogen to polyunsaturated cottonseed oil made it more saturated and turned it into a solid fat at room temperature. If you look on the labels of many manufactured food items you will see the words *partially hydrogenated*—meaning that the manufacturer added hydrogen to a polyunsaturated fat, making it into a trans fat. The more saturated a fat becomes, the stiffer and more solid it gets. Trans fats are also less likely to go rancid and thus have a longer shelf life.

Procter & Gamble used what was abundant and cheap in the early 1900s—cottonseed oil—to build its partially hydrogenated evil twin—Crisco. In the 1930s the same technology was applied to the increasingly cheap and very abundant soybean oil. Today you will see that many oils are subject to this potentially dangerous process, sometimes even olive oil. (Is nothing sacred?)

Cholesterol Free, Partially Hydrogenated, and Dangerous

Fast foods are probably the biggest single source of trans fats in our diet. Up until the late 1980s, fast-food restaurants deep-fried food in beef tallow loaded with artery-choking saturated fats. In the early 1990s McDonalds, responding in part to public pressure,

Worshipping the Golden Arches

When I lived in Rome in the late 1970s there was no McDonalds in the entire city. As far as I knew there was only one in the country, and that was up north in Milan. But things have changed in Italy and throughout the Mediterranean because McDonalds has opened new stores around the globe—at a rate of over 2,000 a year. When I recently returned to Italy, I was chagrined to see a McDonalds planted near the Pantheon. It is a blight on a formerly beautiful piazza and symbolizes an ominous cultural shift to unhealthy foods for Italians and all Mediterraneans.

But placing a McDonalds near the Pantheon has particular significance: In the 1500's the Barberini pope ordered the Pantheon ceiling stripped of its bronze to build the great altar of St. Peter's. This assault on a historic treasure outraged Romans and was immortalized in the Roman saying: "What the barbarians didn't do to Rome, the Barberini did." Italian cuisine, like the Pantheon and the Pieta, is one of that culture's most valuable treasures. Today a force more powerful than the barbarians or the Barberini is threatening that treasure. It is the dietary, anti-culture represented by the Golden Arches.

proudly announced that its fries would be cooked in "Cholesterol-free 100 percent vegetable oil." While this is true, it was not the whole truth. The whole truth is that McDonalds uses partially hydrogenated vegetable oil. In other words, it uses trans fats, which are at least as bad for your blood cholesterol as the saturated fats they replaced, and probably worse. In some ways this is another kind of high-fat fraud. You go into McDonalds and choose the fries instead of the burger, thinking you're avoiding saturated fat. But it turns out that you're no better off, because the fries are loaded with trans fats. But what's truly frightening is the way they are fried. Temperatures used for deep-frying liberate legions of deadly free radicals from fats. But even more frightening is the effect of multiple frying episodes. Fats that are used again and again for frying oxidize at frighteningly high rates. The next time you see a basket of fries plunged into a vat of bubbling brown oil, you should get out of that place as quickly as possible. (By the way, virgin olive oil is remarkably resistant to oxidation even after multiple frying episodes.) And don't be seduced into thinking that the chicken-based fast foods are healthier than the burger alternatives. McDonalds Chicken McNuggets, Burger King's Chicken Sandwich, Boston Market's Chicken Pot Pie, and KFC's Original Recipe Dinner are all loaded with trans fats. They are like nutritional Trojan horses that sneak trans fats into your body. Real Greeks would never eat this stuff. They would use them only as gifts for their enemies. For real Greeks the fat of choice is olive oil.

11 Fraud Foods

While fast foods are the biggest source of trans fats, trans fats are put in many foods that are marketed as low-fat, low-cholesterol, or "healthy." Despite the danger these foods present to our health, manufacturers love trans fats because they're cheaper than other solid fats and give foods a fuller taste than pure polyunsaturated fats. They also have a longer shelf life than the polyunsaturated fats they are made from and they enable manufacturers to use the food marketing phrases: "cholesterol free" and "no saturated fat." To find these furtive fats in foods, you can't just read the nutrition facts label that lists calories and percentages of fat and carbohydrates. You have to read the small print under "Ingredients." There you will find a reference to partially hydrogenated oil—usually soybean, cottonseed, or canola oil. That's your trans fat.

Trans fats combine the worst features of saturated fats and polyunsaturated fats. Like saturated fats, trans fats raise LDL levels,

> ### "Spreading" Death
>
> Margarine spreads were supposed to be our salvation from heart disease, but they often contain trans fats, which increase the risk of heart disease. In fact, solid margarine may cause more heart disease than the butter it was supposed to replace. Like a nutritional Trojan horse, some food manufacturers put trans fats into their foods but still claim their product is a gift to your health. One should be wary of food manufacturers bearing gifts. If you see "partially hydrogenated" oil on the label, stay away.

and like polyunsaturated fats, they lower HDL levels. From what we know about blood cholesterol, nothing could be worse for your health. While trans fats constitute only a small fraction of the American diet, it seems that trans fats are poisons that may be responsible for a great deal of heart disease. In the Nurses' Health Study, women who consumed the highest amounts of trans fats had an 80 percent higher risk of heart attacks compared to women who consumed the lowest amounts of trans fats.

An Unhealthy Choice

ConAgra is a multibillion-dollar food manufacturing behemoth. From Wesson oil to Armour meats to Healthy Choice meals, it manufactures more products than you can imagine. The Healthy Choice line is a direct response to the call for lower-fat foods. Low in saturated fat and low in cholesterol, the meals are clearly presented as a heart-healthy line of foods. The problem is that they are laced with trans fats. There are scores of Healthy Choice products ranging from puddings to dinners; virtually every one we checked had partially hydrogenated fats or trans fats in it. So even though these products are low in cholesterol and saturated fat, they contain a substance that, even in small amounts, may do more harm to your blood cholesterol levels than consuming cholesterol or saturated fat.

While the amount of trans fats in Healthy Choice meals is very small, they are everywhere in very small amounts. Snackwells cookies and most of Nabisco's snack-food line, including its supposedly heart-healthy, reduced-fat products like reduced-fat Oreos and Chips Ahoy, all have trans fats. Trans fats are even in Nabisco's Zwieback cookies for babies. The Keebler elves are no better; they stuff trans fats in almost every cookie they make. You would think rice cakes would be safe, but no, trans fats are in Orville Redenbacher's caramel rice cakes.

> Of the physicians responding to our survey, a shocking 69 percent did not know trans-fatty acids raised LDL, or bad cholesterol, levels. A whopping 80 percent did not know that trans-fatty acids would lower HDL, or good cholesterol, levels.

Trans fats are not only in baked goods; Pizza Hut's pizza sauce, Jif and Skippy peanut butters (including the reduced-fat peanut butters), and Wishbone Lite Blue Cheese salad dressing all contain trans fats. Doritos WOW chips appeal to your health consciousness by proclaiming to be low in fat, but they have both olestra and trans fats—a double whammy. Nabisco and ConAgra may say that the small amount of trans fats in a single Snackwells cookie or Healthy Choice meal every now and then isn't going to kill you. That's true. However, hydrogenated fats are all around us in small amounts, and they add up. For example, take a look at this list of trans-fat foods with labels that would lead you to believe they are healthy:

Trans Fat Travesties

Trans fats are put in foods that are marketed as low-fat, low-cholesterol, or "healthy." We've listed some of these trans fat–filled "healthy" foods. The nutrients are listed relative to their content—if partially hydrogenated fats are listed before vegetables, for instance, then there are more hydrogenated fats by weight than vegetables in the product.

Healthy Choice:

Herb baked fish—Partially hydrogenated soybean and cottonseed oil are listed after fish and before vegetables.

Grilled chicken Sonoma—Partially hydrogenated cottonseed and soybean oil are in the onions and the roasted tomato flavor.

Macaroni and cheese—Partially hydrogenated oils, including soybean and cottonseed oils, are listed three times, including after the cheese flavor and in the margarine.

Chicken fettuccine Alfredo—Contains partially hydrogenated soybean oil.

Tuna casserole—Partially hydrogenated soybean oil is listed four times, including in the bread crumbs, butter flavor, and the margarine.

Supreme French bread pizza—Contains vegetable shortening that has partially hydrogenated soybean and cottonseed oils.

Cappuccino mocha fudge brownie premium low-fat ice cream—Contains coconut oil, and partially hydrogenated cottonseed and soybean oils are in the cake bits.

Weight Watchers:

Lemon-herb chicken Piccata—Contains partially hydrogenated soybean oil.

Honey mustard chicken—Contains partially hydrogenated soybean oil in margarine and in beef flavor.

Orville Redenbacher's caramel popcorn cakes—Contain partially hydrogenated soybean oil.

Frito Lay WOW brand Doritos tortilla chips—Olestra is the second ingredient; the chips also contain partially hydrogenated cottonseed and soybean oils.

Snackwells:

Creme sandwich cookies—Contain partially hydrogenated canola, soybean, and/or cottonseed oils.

Double chocolate chip cookies—Contain vegetable shortening with partially hydrogenated soybean oil.

Peanut butter chip cookies—The chips contain partially hydrogenated soybean and cottonseed oils; the peanut butter contains hydrogenated rapeseed, cottonseed, and soybean oils.

Devil's food cookies—Contain vegetable shortening and partially hydrogenated soybean oil.

Zesty cheese crackers—Contain partially hydrogenated soybean oil and/or soybean oil.

Wheat crackers—Contain partially hydrogenated soybean oil and/or soybean oil.

Cracked pepper crackers—Contain soybean oil and/or partially hydrogenated canola oil.

Trans Fats in Nabisco Foods

- 5 Grain Harvest Crisps (label says 55 percent less fat)
- Arrowroot (label says, "Babies' first cookie for over 100 years")
- Cameo (label says low cholesterol)
- Cheese Nips Reduced Fat
- Chips Ahoy Reduced Fat
- Low-fat Graham Crackers
- Nabisco Better Cheddars Reduced Fat
- Nilla Wafers Reduced Fat
- Nutter Butter (label says low cholesterol)
- Oreos Reduced Fat
- Ritz Reduced Fat
- Saltines (label says, "No Cholesterol and Low in Saturated Fat")
- Social Tea (label says low cholesterol, low saturated fat)
- Triscuits Reduced Fat
- Wheat Thins Reduced Fat (label says whole wheat)
- Zwieback (label says, "Over a century of wholesome goodness")

The Small Amounts May Be Killing Us

In the beginning of the twentieth century trans fats were unknown in the American diet. Today they represent 3 to 5 percent of calories. Their growing use since first introduced in 1911 closely tracks the steep rise in heart disease in the United States. In fact, trans fats track this rise more closely than even saturated fats, which have been steadily declining as a percentage of calories consumed. Dr. Martin Katan, the internationally famous lipid researcher from the Netherlands, found that replacing only 2 percent of saturated fats with trans fats produced a dramatic worsening of the LDL-HDL ratio. This suggests that not only do tiny quantities of trans fats dramatically increase the risk of heart disease, but they seem to be even more dangerous than the much-dreaded saturated fats.

Remember, the olive oil–rich Mediterranean diet contains virtually no trans fats. It is a much healthier choice than Healthy Choice meals from ConAgra.

Part Two:
Good News from the Mediterranean

12 The Healthiest Diet in the World

With all the rhetoric about the importance of low-fat diets, you would think that the healthiest cultures consumed the least fat. But the healthiest diet in the world, or at the very least the Western world, contains 40 percent fat. It is the diet traditionally consumed on the Greek Island of Crete. In the early 1950s researcher Leland Albaugh described the Cretan diet this way: "Olives, cereal grains, pulses [legumes], wild greens, and herbs and fruits together with limited quantities of goat meat and milk, game and fish have remained the basic Cretan foods for forty centuries.... No meal was complete without bread.... Olives and olive oil contributed significantly to energy intake.... Food seemed literally to be 'swimming' in oil."

Swimming in oil! That's enough to make any low-fat fanatic freak out. Nevertheless, the health benefits of this Cretan-Greek diet are well documented. In 1961, census data on Greece revealed that despite widespread smoking, rampant poverty, high childhood mortality rates, and poor health care, the life expectancy of Greek adults was higher than any other national group tracked by the World Health Organization. The recognition that Greece and other Mediterranean countries like Italy had dramatically lower rates of heart disease provided the impetus for landmark research linking diet and disease.

At a 1952 nutrition conference in Rome, nutrition researcher Dr. Ancel Keys noted the new epidemic of coronary artery disease that was rampant in the United States and parts of Europe. Dr. Gino Bergami, professor of physiology at the University of Naples, responded that there was no such epidemic in Naples. Keys went to sunny Naples to take a closer look. In this southern Italian city, originally named Neopolis by the Greeks who had settled it thousands of years before, Keys found that heart attacks were indeed rare except among the upper classes, who consumed more meat than other Neapolitans. His wife Margaret measured cholesterol levels and found that they were low except among members of the Neapolitan Rotary club—the same upper-class people who were suffering what few heart attacks occurred in Naples.

The low heart-disease rates in Naples, high rates in Northern Europe and America, and connections to blood cholesterol and diet stimulated Keys to begin the large-scale Seven Country Study. This study was an enormous undertaking that sought to find associations between heart disease, diet, and death in seven different countries. Its findings strongly influenced nutrition policy for the remainder of the century.

Beginning in the late 1950s Keys and his colleagues amassed mountains of data on more than twelve thousand men from seven countries—Finland, Greece, Italy, Japan, Yugoslavia, the Netherlands, and the United States. They studied fifteen different groups

Spain, Olive Oil, and Longevity

A report published in 1998 reveals that Spain, the world's largest producer of olive oil and one of its largest consumers, now has the greatest life expectancy in the Western world—78 years for men and 81.1 for women.

of men, each group five hundred to one thousand in numbe. They found that the lowest rates of death, cancer, and heart disease were on the Greek islands of Crete and Corfu, in other Mediterranean sites, and in Japan. Among these, the Cretans had the lowest rates of heart disease and cancer, and the lowest death rates.

Despite the unhealthy effects of poverty, poor medical care, and high rates of smoking, the Cretans achieved a level of health the American Heart Association, the National Cancer Institute, and the National Cholesterol Education Program can only dream about; and they achieved it on a high-fat diet that exceeded these agencies' maximum threshold for fat by at least 33 percent. Keys called these healthy diets from southern Europe the "good Mediterranean diet."

The study followed up on the participants at five-year intervals to see how many had died, or had contracted cancer or heart disease. *In 1984 a fifteen-year analysis was published, revealing that the Cretans had lower rates of heart disease and death than even the Japanese.* In fact the men from Japan had twice the overall death rate as the men from Crete, and even though the Japanese were famous for incredibly low rates of heart disease, their heart disease rates were still almost four times those of Cretan men.

It was also clear from this study that all Mediterranean diets are not equal. Even though countries like Italy and France are Mediterranean, there is tremendous variation in the diets consumed throughout these countries. As you go farther north in Italy and France, more meat and saturated fat are consumed and the rates of heart disease go up. As you head south in these countries, meat consumption goes down and olive oil consumption goes up, more resembling the Cretan diet. The more these diets resemble the traditional Cretan diet, steeped in vegetables, olive oil, and red wine, the healthier people are.

Not only did the Seven Country Study demonstrate the remarkable health benefits of the Mediterranean diet, it also convincingly demonstrated a tight association among blood cholesterol, saturated fat, heart disease, and premature death. Unfortunately, the breakthrough identification of saturated fat as a key villain in heart disease was distorted by a subsequent obsession with eliminating almost all fat. Instead of looking further into the positive benefits of monounsaturated fat—found in olive oil—nutrition leaders (including Keys at first) advocated polyunsaturated fats like corn and safflower oils, and partially hydrogenated margarines.

One reason is that in those days they could test only for total blood cholesterol. The technology to measure both LDL and HDL had not yet been developed. It was found that while polyunsaturated fat lowered total cholesterol under experimental conditions, monounsaturated fat did not. And so it was assumed that polyunsaturated fats were superior. What they did not know, of course, is that both monounsaturated and polyunsaturated fat lowered LDL levels, but monounsaturated fat maintained or raised HDL levels. So even though monounsaturated fat was reducing LDL levels, it did not reduce total levels of cholesterol because it was also raising HDL levels. Despite the central role of olive oil and monounsaturated fat in the Mediterranean diet, it was lost in the translation to an American diet.

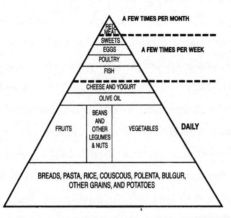

A FEW TIMES PER MONTH

RED MEAT

SWEETS

EGGS   A FEW TIMES PER WEEK

POULTRY

FISH

CHEESE AND YOGURT

OLIVE OIL

FRUITS | BEANS AND OTHER LEGUMES & NUTS | VEGETABLES | DAILY

BREADS, PASTA, RICE, COUSCOUS, POLENTA, BULGUR, OTHER GRAINS, AND POTATOES

The Mediterranean Diet pyramid was developed by Oldways Preservation and Exchange Trust and is a valuable contribution to nutrition education. Unlike the U.S. Department of Agriculture pyramid, which was influenced by the meat lobby, the Mediterranean pyramid is extremely healthy. This is the pyramid that should be hanging in doctors' offices and classrooms.

In 1986 another follow-up analysis of the Seven Country Study was published, and it revealed that a high ratio of monounsaturated to saturated fat was the best predictor of health. In other words, high intakes of monounsaturated fat and low intakes of saturated fat were associated with lower rates of heart disease, cancer, and overall death. It was now clear that olive oil played a central role in making the Cretan-Mediterranean diet perhaps the healthiest diet in the world. Unfortunately, by this time the low-fat lies were well entrenched.

In the past fifty years traditional ways of eating, in Crete and throughout the Mediterranean, have changed due to increasing affluence and the "McDonaldization" of the world. Yet Cretans and other Mediterraneans who cling to the old ways of eating remain healthy and enjoy continued protection against the diseases of modern life. For instance, women of Toulouse in southern France who still consume a healthy Mediterranean diet rich in vegetables and olive oil rival Japanese women for being the longest-living people and having the lowest rates of heart disease. Spaniards as a whole are second, by a fraction, to the Japanese in total longevity. Dr. Antonia Trichopoulou studied the dietary habits of 182 Greek men and women over the age of seventy and found that those who departed from the traditional diet, primarily by eating more meat and less beans, had a significantly higher risk of death over a period of five years. But those who stuck to the traditional Greek diet had significantly lower death rates.

How Do We Know It's Not the Dancing?

Dr. Henry Blackburn, a world-famous expert on nutrition from Minnesota and a collaborator in the Seven Country Study, described Cretan life:

> The Cretan walks to work daily and labors in the soft light of his Greek isle... in the peace of his land. At the end of the morning's work, he rests and socializes with cohorts at the local cafe.... He continues the siesta with a meal and a nap at home.... The ritual family dinner is followed by relaxing fellowship with peers... Festivity builds to a passionate midnight dance.... He is secure in his niche... relishes the natural rhythmic cycles and contrasts of his culture.... The greatest life expectancy in the western world.

Nikos Kazantzakis, a Cretan who wrote *Zorba the Greek* long before Anthony Quinn immortalized the role, could not have described it any better. But how do we know it's the diet that gives Zorba his vigor and his remarkable longevity? How do we know it's not the dancing? After all, in the Keys study the cholesterol levels in Crete

The Traditional Mediterranean Diet

The following is Dr. Ancel Keys's observations while studying the traditional diet of southern Italians:

> Homemade minestrone... pasta in an endless variety... served with tomato sauce and a sprinkle of cheese, only occasionally enriched with some bits of meat, or served with a little local seafood... a hearty dish of beans and short lengths of macaroni... lots of bread never more than a few hours from the oven and never served with any kind of spread; great quantities of fresh vegetables; a modest portion of meat or fish perhaps twice a week; always fresh fruit for dessert.... Years later, when called on to devise diets for the possible prevention of coronary disease, we looked back and concluded that it would be hard to do better than to imitate the diet of the common folk of Naples in the early 1950s.

Although Keys described the essence of the southern Italian diet, he does make the conspicuous error of overlooking olive oil. This is an oversight that undermined some of his early recommendations about diet.

weren't much different from those in other Mediterranean populations, yet Cretan men had substantially lower rates of heart disease.

The Cretan lifestyle is important, but if we separate diet from dancing and other factors, we can see just how important diet is. Recently a group of French doctors from the University of Lyon led by Dr. Serge Renaud conducted such an experiment to evaluate the effectiveness of a Cretan-like diet in preventing heart disease.

The Cretan Diet in France

The French have confounded the experts for years because they have relatively low rates of heart disease despite relatively high national intakes of saturated fats. This "French Paradox," as Dr. Renaud first called it, has been explained in a variety of ways. Some, such as Renaud, have proposed that the high intake of red wine is protective (and it probably is). Others have proposed that getting your saturated fat from cheese is not quite as bad as getting it from meat, and there seems to be something to this as well. Others have prointed out that the French who live in the north and have the highest intakes of saturated fats die younger than their olive oil–consuming, Mediterranean countrymen in the south. That's true too. Despite the unresolved controversy, French heart patients are routinely put on a diet that is considered prudent for their condition—a diet that is similar to the one recommended by the American Heart Association (AHA). Aware of the longevity of Cretans the researchers from Lyon set out to discover if the Cretan diet was superior to the diet they were prescribing for their patients. They gathered approximately six hundred French heart patients; half went on the Cretan-like diet, and the other half went on the traditional heart-healthy diet. Those on the Cretan diet, which is very rich in monounsaturated fat, were given a special spread made with canola oil. They also used olive oil for salads and food preparation.

The remarkable benefits of the Cretan diet were seen after only twenty-seven months. Although both groups consumed the same quantity of total fat, the group eating the Cretan monounsaturated fat diet had 70 to 80 percent fewer heart-related problems—from chest pains to heart attacks—and a 70 percent lower rate of overall death compared with the group eating the AHA-type diet.

What made these results even more remarkable was that there was no difference in measurements of cholesterol and triglycerides in the blood. In other words, their blood lipid profiles, traditionally the best indicator we have of heart disease, were essentially the same, and yet there were big differences in the amount of heart disease. How can we explain this?

One answer is that monounsaturated fats, unlike polyunsaturated fats, are resistant to oxidation, and olive oil carries its own supply of antioxidants. This suggests that at a given cholesterol level, less of that cholesterol is likely to be oxidized.

Renaud continued to follow the original participants and published a follow-up report in June 1998. Remarkably, after four years, the people on the Cretan diet had significantly fewer deaths—not only from cardiac disease, but from all causes, including cancer. The patients on the Cretan diet had higher blood levels of both vitamin C and vitamin E, even though they consumed lower quantities of vitamin E. Oxidation and free-radical formation are probably at the heart of this seemingly paradoxical finding. Vitamin E is a powerful antioxidant that is consumed in its battles against the free radicals created by oxidation. Because the Cretan diet is rich in monounsaturated fat, the level of ongoing oxidation is probably more limited, and less vitamin E may be consumed.

The shocking bottom line is that a diet rich in monounsaturated fat may be superior to the traditional heart-healthy diet prescribed by many physicians around the world. Furthermore, it seems to promote high circulating levels of vitamin E and other antioxidants that may help prevent heart disease as well as certain kinds of cancer. Ultimately it shows that Cretan longevity is not just the result of the dancing; it's also the diet.

The Healthiest Diet in the Eastern World

The low-fat diet of the Japanese has been the inspiration for many who advocate low-fat diets. In Keys's study the Japanese were second only to the Cretans in rates of heart disease and death, and for decades the Japanese have topped the charts in national longevity tables. So why do we keep harping on the importance of fat when the Japanese eat an extremely low-fat diet and do just fine?

As one might expect, the traditional Mediterranean and Japanese diets share some common features. Both are low in saturated fat, polyunsaturated fat, and trans-fatty acids. Both have low intakes of red meat and high intakes of grains, legumes, vegetables, and other plant-based foods. But while the Cretans consume large quantities of fruits and no seaweed, the Japanese consume little fruit and large amounts of seaweed (if you think it's hard to get kids to eat peas, try seaweed). And while the Japanese consume almost no monounsaturated fat, they do consume enormous quantities of fish and fish oil, containing the extremely healthy omega-3 fatty acids. The Cretans get their dose of omega-3 fatty acids through nuts, and both diets include regular alcohol consumption, although the Cretans consume more red wine. The Japanese consume more soy, which is endowed with many health-promoting phytochemicals and may be more relevant to their health than how much total fat they consume.

There is no question that the classic Japanese diet is a healthy diet, and along with a vigorous exercise program, it will, like the Mediterranean diet, do wonders for your health. Yet for many if not most Americans, the Mediterranean approach offers more promise.

First, Keys studied Japanese farming and fishing villages. Only about 6 percent of those studied were considered sedentary, while almost twice as many Cretans and 10 times as many Americans were considered sedentary when the Keys study was done in the 1960s. You will recall that the best defense against low HDL cholesterol and high triglycerides that come with low-fat, high-carbohydrate diets is vigorous, consistent exercise. While a low-fat, high-carbohydrate diet might be fine for Japanese fishermen, it is frequently the wrong prescription for many sedentary Americans. In a couch-potato country where the metabolic syndrome—obesity, hypertension, low HDL, high triglycerides, small LDL, increased blood-clotting tendencies, and elevated insulin—is epidemic, low-fat diets that don't result in weight loss may make matters worse for many.

There is good evidence that many American palates will rebel against a diet that almost completely excludes fat, making it difficult to adhere to this diet for a lifetime. We know from studies like one published in the *Journal of the American Medical Association* in 1997 that it is difficult for even highly motivated Americans to consume a diet that is less than 20 percent fat for extended lengths of time. In this study of 440 highly motivated men, those aiming to stick to a diet containing 18 percent of calories from fat for a year could get down to only 22 percent, and those aiming for 22 percent could get down to only 25 percent. Meanwhile, those aiming for a more reasonable 30 percent were more successful and also avoided the rising tide of triglycerides that is frequently triggered when a diet drops below 25 percent of calories from fat. Also there was no difference in weight loss between those who consumed a higher percentage of fat and those who consumed a lower percentage. Staying below 10 percent or even 20 percent of calories from fat is wildly unrealistic for most Americans. The fat content of the healthy Mediterranean diet, which is mostly in a range between 28 and 38 percent of calories from fat, seems more achievable and sustainable for most Americans.

The Japanese diet is a wonderful diet, and it works. But properly simulating the diet means purchasing, preparing, and consuming foods that are perhaps more foreign to many Americans who are not of Japanese or Asian descent. It means consuming very large quantities of fish, a problem in a culture in which frequent shopping for fresh fish is not often practical. It also means consuming large quantities of soy and seaweed. This is not to say it can't be done, but it's a bit more of a challenge for many Americans. Some might object that olive oil and the Mediterranean diet may be foreign to many Americans. This is true, but it is a question of degree. For most Americans, the Mediterranean diet is relatively more familiar, more universal, and more achievable.

The Japanese diet is not a low-fat or no-fat diet in the same way that Americans interpret that phrase. Their manner of eating isn't dictated by some narrow obsession with eliminating a certain kind of nutrient. Like all natural and culturally based cuisines, it is food focused. It is a centuries-old way of preparing and eating a diversity of natural foods. As with the Mediterranean diet, the foods stand in relation to each other as members of a symphony and produce a cuisine and a diet that is harmonious not only with the individual foods but with a way of life. It is that harmony, together with the natural rhythms of the culture, that are important to the success of these cuisines over a lifetime. It is difficult to fully recreate this cultural rhythm in a foreign environment, but by at least committing to a type of cuisine we increase our chances of adhering to a diet. It will simply become how we eat and live.

So if you are of Japanese or Asian heritage, or merely love those cuisines, you should embrace them. But remember, to avoid the negative effects of low-fat diets you may need to lose weight, exercise, or both. And if you want to lose weight you still need to limit calories. Eating tofu by the truckload will put on weight just as surely as too much pasta, too much meat, or too much olive oil.

The Healthiest Diet in the World—Japan vs. Crete

So, what's the worlds healthiest diet? It's impossible to say with absolute certainty. Good studies have documented that the traditional Japanese and Cretan diets are two of the healthiest. The Seven Country Study is the best comparison of the Japanese and Cretan diets, even though the data was last analyzed in the 1980s, because it compares these diets in their traditional forms, largely uncorrupted by affluence and American influence. In the Seven Country Study, the Cretan diet was associated with better health and lower death rates than the Japanese diet.

> The MONICA project monitored cardiovascular disease in twenty-seven countries and thirty-eight populations on four continents. The MONICA project paralleled the Seven Country Study in that among the regions studied, those with the lowest rates of coronary heart disease were from the Mediterranean and Asia.

Still, despite the amazing health of the Cretans, the Japanese diet has gotten far more publicity than the Cretan Diet, and many nutrition experts seem to favor it. This is probably because Japan has topped the longevity charts in recent years, edging out Greece and Spain by a whisker, and partly because the Japanese diet fits into their low-fat view of the world. However, Japan's slight longevity edge is in part related to a dramatically low infant-mortality rate and high socioeconomic status. Furthermore, Crete—which is a region, not a country—doesn't appear on these recent

How Lies Get Started

How could clear-cut associations between monounsaturated fat, olive oil, and health be so completely overlooked and so egregiously underemphasized? The message to reduce total fat came through loud and clear. But the message to consume monounsaturated fat has been muted at best. No one intended to lie, but early errors in judgment and unfortunate compromises started us in the wrong direction. The battle for nutritional health somehow got subordinated to a war on fat. And like all wars, it was heavily influenced by politics, power, and money.

According to food reformer Dun Gifford, one of the early skirmishes was fought by President Dwight Eisenhower himself. Dr. Paul Dudley White, who had written a heart-healthy cookbook with Ancel Keys based on the results of Keys's Seven Country Study, told Eisenhower that he had to give up beef and eat more like the Mediterraneans. Eisenhower reportedly refused, claiming that an American president couldn't do something as un-American as giving up steak. White informed him that if he didn't change his diet and eat less meat, he would soon be a dead president. Eisenhower compromised, agreeing to eat a Mediterranean-style, plant-based diet on the condition that it be kept a secret. Ike dissembled about his diet because he knew that food was a political issue.

By the 1970s science had caught up with red meat and saturated fat. The Senate Select Committee on Nutrition and Human Needs, chaired by Senator George McGovern, held hearings on the connections between food and chronic disease and in 1977 issued a report that contained the first federal dietary recommendations for the prevention of chronic disease. To achieve its goals the committee recommended, among other things, a reduction in the consumption of meat. This was a sound, food-based guideline that was easy to understand. Unfortunately it provoked an uproar from the meat industry and its lobbyists. So the committee revised its first report and issued a second edition. Instead of calling for a "decrease in the consumption of meat," the compromise statement was altered to emphasize avoidance of certain nutrients—that is, fats—rather than specific foods such as meat. The new wording read, "Decrease consumption of animal fat, and choose meats, poultry, and fish which will reduce saturated fat intake." Rather than casting meat in a negative light, this seemed to encourage meat consumption. One might even interpret it as proclaiming that red meats can reduce saturated fat. *But the most enduring and damaging effect was to shift the emphasis from food-based guidelines to nutrient-based guidelines, and fat—all fat—became public enemy number one.* The committee, ignoring the evidence provided by healthy Greek peasants—vigorous, real-life Zorbas who consumed diets that were almost 40 percent fat—recommended that all Americans consume diets with 30 percent fat or less. There were no population data or experimental data to suggest that there was anything special about a 30 percent threshold. It was an arbitrary choice. Nonetheless it has been a national goal ever since. And, by the way, the national obesity epidemic started in the 1970s.

World Health Organization longevity charts, which show only national rates.

There are definite benefits to the Japanese diet when compared to the standard American diet, but it does have some drawbacks. Over the years the national data from Japan reveal excessively high rates of stroke possibly due to extremely low cholesterol levels or extremely low-fat diets. Japan also has disproportionately high cancer rates, which may be related to extremely high levels of cooked fish intake or low levels of fruit consumption. The Japanese diet in fact may not be, to the surprise of many, the healthiest diet in the world. The honor may go to the traditional Cretan diet, a diet that ranges between 38 and 42 percent fat. Hard for fat phobes to believe. But true.

13 Nature's Healthiest Oil

From the dawn of recorded time, olive oil has been the cornerstone of the Mediterranean diet. Some written records referring to olive oil are at least six thousand years old. Olive oil and olives, along with bread and wine, are the most frequently mentioned foods in the Bible (one might even say it's God's oil). The olive branch became an immortal symbol of hope and life when a dove brought one back to Noah's ark after the Great Flood. The olive tree itself suggests immortality by its capacity to live hundreds of years. Some say there are olive trees that have lived a thousand years. For the Greeks, the olive tree, a gift from Athena, became the symbol of immortality when it regenerated itself after the enemies of Athens razed the city and burned their sacred tree to a stump. Little could those Greeks have known that many centuries later, the oil of that tree would make them famous—if not for their immortality, then at least for their remarkable longevity.

The esteem ancient peoples placed in this tree and its fruit was a testament to the remarkable contribution it made to their lives. Olive oil was (and is) a valuable source of calories and a crucial element in their delicious cuisine. It could also be burned in lanterns to produce light. The oil warded off hunger and darkness; it would have been hard for these ancient people to imagine life without it. It was, and we believe it remains, the oil of life.

Virginity, when applied to olive oil, refers to the purity of the oil as well as the way it was produced. Olive oil remains the only commonly used oil that can be mass-produced in a completely organic, unprocessed way. Corn kernels, safflower seeds, soybeans, and rapeseed plants do not easily give up their oils and must be subjected to a variety of processes to yield their fats. The juicy olive is merely pressed, much like grapes for wine, and its life-preserving oil flows freely, as if nature had designed the fruit for this purpose. After most of the oil has been pressed out, the debris that is left behind can be coaxed to give up some more oil if hot water and further intense pressure is added, but this second hot pressing produces an oil that is inferior in taste and quality. Today almost all mass-produced olive oil for human consumption comes from the first, cold pressing.

Virgin olive oil not only must be cold-pressed, but it must also have measurable acidity between 1 and 3.3 percent. Extra-virgin olive oil must have less than 1 percent measurable acidity. Both virgin and extra-virgin olive oils must also have excellent aroma, flavor, and color. Olive oil that does not carry the label "virgin" or "extra virgin" is a combination of refined, processed olive oil and virgin oil. Some batches of oil have to be refined because inferior olives were used. The refined oil has no taste or smell, and virgin oil is added to give it flavor. The less virgin oil that is added, the

Fruits, Vegetables, Olive Oil

Olive oil contains a number of phytochemicals—such as caffeic acid, vanillic acid, and oleuropein—that seem to promote the production and limit the destruction of nitric oxide (NO), a crucial heart attack–preventing compound manufactured by the body. Moreover, some of the other foods in the Mediterranean diet also seem to protect NO and promote its production. The Mediterranean diet is extraordinarily rich in fruits and vegetables. These plants supply a wealth of phytochemicals and antioxidants that also help prevent injury to the walls of the coronary arteries. They help prevent the oxidation of LDL cholesterol and provide other substances that help promote NO production. A bit of fat is necessary to absorb some phytochemicals, such as carotenes, and get the maximum benefit from them. Of course, plants are also a very rich source of fiber.

less flavor the resulting oil has. Oils called simply "olive oil" must still have an acidity of not more than 1.5 percent. Because generic olive oil is cheaper than virgin or extra virgin olive oil, it is often used for cooking. However, while still a monounsaturated fat, it is not clear how many phytochemicals and other health-promoting substances are lost in the refined, processed variety of olive oil.

When you use virgin and extra-virgin olive oil you can be certain that you are using very pure, high-quality, unprocessed, unrefined oil. Naturally occurring foods dressed and enhanced with a naturally occurring oil are vital in the struggle to maintain health in the modern world. Let's face it—Snackwells; Big Macs; Pringles; Pepsi; and foods containing highly processed, partially hydrogenated corn, safflower, or soybean oil are not what nature had in mind for us to live on.

There is a popular myth that olive oil is not useful for cooking at high temperatures. While it is true that olive oil has a lower smoke point than polyunsaturated fats like corn oil or soybean oil, olive oil doesn't begin to smoke until about 400 degrees Fahrenheit. It would be unusual for home cooking or frying to exceed that temperature. In fact, olive oil is far superior for frying and sautéing at home. That's because the tendency for polyunsaturated fats to oxidize is greatly magnified when they are heated. In some cases, the speed of oxidation has been reported to be one hundred times that of olive oil. That makes some polyunsaturated fats, like those containing otherwise healthy omega-3 fatty acids, potentially dangerous when they are used for frying. It gets even worse when polyunsaturated fats are used for repeated frying, as often happens in commercial or fast-food environments.

Throughout this book we have referred to the benefits of monounsaturated fats as well as the phytochemicals in olive oil. But the phytochemicals and other micronutrients in olive oil have remained mysterious entities that have, by and large, lacked names or detailed descriptions. This is mostly because these substances are just being discovered. What is known is largely based on animal research and needs to be verified in humans. Still we thought it would be important to list a few of the more than two hundred phytochemicals and micronutrients found in olive oil and briefly describe what is known about them so far.

Phytochemicals and Micronutrients

Caffeic acid. Caffeic acid has been shown to be a very effective antioxidant. There is evidence that caffeic acid works with vitamin E to prevent LDL oxidation. Caffeic acid has also been shown to stop the production of potential cancer-causing compounds that form when meat is cooked. Other research has shown that caffeic acid not only blocks carcinogens from attacking cells but also inhibits tumor growth once a cancerous process has started. But that's not all. Caffeic acid has been shown to inhibit the growth of some bacteria and fungi and also to inhibit xanthine oxidase, the enzyme that makes uric acid. Uric acid is related to the development of gout. This means caffeic acid may play a role in the prevention of cancer and heart disease as well as infections and gout, though these benefits have not yet been verified in humans.

Ferulic acid. Ferulic acid may be even better at preventing LDL oxidation than vitamin C is. It can protect a certain LDL protein from oxidation, thereby decreasing the risk of heart disease. Ferulic acid is also useful in several biochemical reactions that prevent the formation or activity of carcinogens.

Hydroxytyrosol. Hydroxytyrosol has been shown to be a powerful antioxidant that rivals and may even surpass vitamin E in efficacy, suggesting a possible role in preventing cancer and heart disease. It seems to not only prevent the formation of free radicals, but also trap and destroy free radicals if they do form. It also prevents platelets from aggregating and forming clots. This latter property may play a role in preventing heart disease.

Oleuropein. Oleuropein has been shown to protect LDL from oxidation and to inhibit the growth of some bacteria and fungi. Oleuropein has anti-inflammatory properties, which suggests that it might play a role in inhibiting damaging inflammation in arteries. Other studies have shown that oleuropein enhances the production of nitric oxide and so may help dilate coronary arteries and improve blood flow to the heart. It is responsible for the bitter taste of olives.

Squalene. Squalene is a rather remarkable compound that is also found in the livers of very-deep-sea fish such as certain rare small sharks. Some believe squalene contributes to the capacity of these fish to survive in such deprived environments in part because it combines easily with oxygen and is useful to tissues when oxygen is in short supply. It has been used in both traditional and alternative medicine in many Eastern countries, particularly Japan and Korea. Although good data are sparse, squalene has been used to treat heart disease and elevated cholesterol, among other conditions. In humans, squalene can be used to make vitamin D or cholesterol. When we are exposed to sun, squalene is made into vitamin D rather than cholesterol. Some feel that this is why cholesterol levels are lower in the summer. There is clearly a great deal more we need to learn about this fascinating compound before we make any definitive claims about its dietary role in human health and disease, but it is very interesting that it is found in olive oil.

Vanillic acid. Vanillic acid is in a class of compounds called polyphenols, which are found in both olive oil and wine. Vanillic acid has been shown to inhibit the growth of some bacteria and fungi, which suggests that it may play a role in fighting infection.

Vitamin E. A fat-soluble vitamin and antioxidant, vitamin E can protect LDL cholesterol from oxidizing, and in some studies it has been associated with lower rates of heart disease. The type of vitamin E that is in olive oil, alpha-tocopherol, is the one that is most easily used by the body. Vitamin E seems to work particularly well with vitamin C, a water-soluble vitamin.

This is a short list of the phytochemicals and micronutrients found in olive oil, but it can give you an idea of why olive oil may be important not only in the prevention of cancer and heart disease but other diseases as well. No doubt future studies will uncover hundreds of other substances that may be just as important. Some studies suggest that olive oil may even prevent diseases other than

More Than Just Monounsaturated Fat

Olive oil contains more than two hundred micronutrients. Some experts think these micronutrients may be even more important than monounsaturated fat when it comes to preventing heart disease. For instance, olive oil is a particularly good source of vitamin E, which has been shown in multiple studies to be associated with lower rates of heart disease.

cancer and heart disease. While one study does not constitute proof by any means, the following are testimony that the role of olive oil may be much more comprehensive than we once thought.

Osteoporosis. In 1997 a study was published suggesting that olive oil may play a role in preventing osteoporosis, possibly by helping the body make vitamin D. Vitamin D plays an important role in calcium absorption, which strengthens bones.

Cataracts. In a study done in northern Italy, it was found that those who consumed more olive oil were less prone to developing cataracts. This is not surprising, because carotenes are known to play a role in lowering the risk of cataracts, and olive oil helps the body absorb carotenes. However, olive oil itself may be reducing the burden of oxidation.

Arthritis. In Greece a study revealed that those who consumed more olive oil were less likely to develop rheumatoid arthritis. Multiple studies have shown a relationship between excessive oxidation and rheumatoid arthritis.

Gallbladder disease. Human experiments suggest that olive oil helps the gallbladder contract more efficiently, thereby promoting easier digestion of fats. Animal research suggests that the monounsaturated fat found in olive oil reduces gallstone forma-

The Secret of Longevity?

In 1965, when Mademoiselle Jeanne Calment was ninety, a shrewd French lawyer began paying her the equivalent of about $500 a month so that he would have first dibs on her choice apartment when she died—not an uncommon arrangement in a tight French housing market. He paid his money each month and rubbed his hands as he eagerly awaited the day when she would move on to the next world and he would move in. He waited a year, then two. But still he did not lose patience. After all, by now she was ninety-two. How much longer could she hang on? Well, ten years passed, and then another ten. And then finally, at long last, death came to the lawyer. Jeanne Calment went on to live to be 123 years old, making her the world's oldest living human when she died in 1997. By the time she finally left this world and

tion. This is supported by studies on humans that show a lower level of gallstone formation in Italian regions where olive oil is more avidly consumed.

Hypertension. There are several studies showing that a diet rich in monounsaturated fats is associated with lower blood pressure. One might speculate that some of the phytochemicals in olive oil that promote nitric oxide production may promote dilation of blood vessels, which, in turn, contributes to lower blood pressure.

Stroke. Recent information based on the Framingham Heart Study suggests that low-fat diets may increase the risk of stroke, while higher-fat diets may be protective. The two most protective fats in the study were monounsaturated fats and saturated fats. Saturated fats, of course, still carry a risk of heart disease and are not recommended.

Aging. While no one has yet discovered an elixir of youth, and

her cherished, highly profitable apartment, Mademoiselle Calment had become world famous and was besieged with
reporters who wanted to know the secret of her longevity. She
told them all the same thing: olive oil and wine.

While we love to hear the advice of our venerable seniors, we
often dismiss it as quickly as we hear it. But in this case that
would be a mistake, because, as science is finally documenting,
Mademoiselle Calment was undoubtedly on to something. Olive
oil and wine are the two pillars upon which the edifice of the
Mediterranean diet rests. They bring not only taste, joy, serenity,
and depth to this diet, but also an extraordinary bounty of chemical substances that promote health and ward off the diseases of
modern life.

while we are not about to claim that olive oil is that elixir, it seems
that oxidation and free-radical formation are important factors in
the aging process. Foods that retard oxidation may slow the aging
process and promote longevity. Olive oil and red wine are two such
foods.

Use Olive Oil to Take Control of Fat

So to use fat to your benefit and take control of the fat in your life,
replace the bad fats in your diet with visible monounsaturated fats
like olive oil. (Canola oil is also a good source of monounsaturated
fat, but olive oil is the basis of the Mediterranean diet.)

Exactly how olive oil will affect you depends on your usual diet.
Let's assume that last week you were on the Standard American
Diet (SAD) of Big Macs, fries, and ice cream, a diet high in satu-
rated fat, carbohydrates, and calories. If you started on a Mediter-

ranean diet this week, keeping total calories the same, within about two weeks you would see a gratifying fall in your LDL cholesterol and triglyceride levels.

Now suppose you weren't on the SAD diet, but a low-fat diet. No Big Macs and not much saturated fat, but lots of carbohydrates and low-fat foods. If you started on a Mediterranean diet, within two weeks you would find that your HDL level would have gone up and your triglyceride level would have gone down and your ratio of small to large LDL might have dropped as well, (overall, your LDL cholesterol level wouldn't change much—it was already pretty low from the low-fat diet).

Another bonus of the olive oil–based Mediterranean diet is that the rest of the foods that make up the diet have very little fat of any kind. The Mediterranean people eat lots of fish and vegetables of every color, plus beans, good breads, and pasta. In fact, it is almost a vegetarian diet, and the vegetables are made palatable by adding olive oil. Mediterranean people use little red meat—they use it almost as a flavoring or condiment—and little butter or milk for adults. Even cheese is used in moderation. As a result the fat in the Mediterranean diet tends to be visible fat— mostly olive oil—which you add to your meals and can precisely measure. That's taking control of the fat in your life.

An American Oil

Some may still see olive oil as foreign to the American culture, but as seen by the evolution of restaurant cuisine in America, olive oil is no longer an exotic item. Though it may seem to be a forbidden fruit to anyone on a low-fat diet, it is no longer seen as strange or foreign. All people who have cultural roots in the biblical tradition—Christians, Jews, or Muslims—have just claim on olive oil

A Fat Worth Fighting For

In an unfortunate chapter of American history, several hundred thousand Italian Americans were put under surveillance and had their personal freedom severely restricted during World War II. About 1,600 Italian citizens living in the United States were shipped off to an internment camp in Missoula, Montana. In a humorous footnote to this largely unknown event, a mini-riot broke out in the camp when the Italian chef was presented with beef fat for frying. His temper got the better of him, and he slapped the American food supplier across the face. Fortunately no one was seriously hurt in the riot that ensued (an American guard shot himself in the foot), but it shows how seriously Italians take their food, and their olive oil. The Italian prisoners knew what modern science is just discovering—that olive oil is vital to good health and longevity. Its virtues are not merely limited to the beneficial monounsaturated fatty acid it contains, oleic acid. The many phytochemicals and micronutrients olive oil contains, which we are just beginning to explore, clearly hold great benefits as well.

as part of their heritage. And when it comes down to it, olive oil is as American as Thomas Jefferson himself, who said, "Of all the gifts of heaven to man, the olive is next to the most precious, if not the most precious." Jefferson advised, "But cover the southern states with olives and every man will become a consumer of oil within whose reach it can be brought in point of price." Sounds like good old Thomas Jefferson, the advocate for the common man, wasn't falling for the low-fat lie.

A Dose of Olive Oil

Think of olive oil as medicine. Certainly, in a world of alternative therapies, it would fit right in. Not only does olive oil have its own beneficial medicinal properties, it has also been shown to enhance the healthful effects of other plant-derived foods. But as with all medicines, olive oil can have side effects. The potential side effect of olive oil is that you may eat too much, which could lead to weight gain. So it is very important to measure olive oil by the teaspoon or tablespoon. But, if used properly, olive oil can be helpful in a weight-loss program. Adding a measured quantity of olive oil to a meal will contribute to satiety, and the fat will help you absorb the fat-soluble nutrients.

On average, a man should consume about 12 teaspoons (or 4 tablespoons) of olive oil a day, or 8 teaspoons (2 1/2 tablespoons) if he is actively pursuing weight loss. An average woman should consume about 8 teaspoons (2 1/2 tablespoons) a day, or 6 teaspoons (2 tablespoons) if she is actively pursuing weight loss. To help you do this, all our recipes are expressed in small amounts of olive oil.

If you don't like thinking of this delicious food as a medicine, think of it as liquid gold or a valuable Mediterranean elixir and watch every drop. Never pour it directly from the bottle. A little bit goes a long way in making food tasty and in contributing to health. Unfortunately, in a lot of low-fat diets, olive oil is forbidden—even in small amounts. This is a major loss in any diet that claims to be a healthy diet.

14 The Truth about Wine

In vino, veritas. In wine, truth. But what is the truth about wine? Well, as we know, absolute proof is hard to come by in matters of nutrition, but the scientific evidence in favor of red wine is especially strong. Multiple comprehensive studies have shown that people who drink alcohol, especially red wine in moderation, live longer and have less heart disease. Other studies have shown exactly *how* wine can prevent disease and prolong life. The evidence is strong enough that people who don't carry obvious risks, like pregnancy, alcoholism, or liver disease, should drink red wine. In fact, physicians should actively advise appropriate patients to drink red wine as part of a treatment plan for preventing heart disease.

The story of wine is as ancient as the olive. By the eighth century B.C., when Homer was composing *The Iliad*, wine was a staple in the Mediterranean diet. The Greek word for breakfast, *akratidzomai*, quite literally means "to drink undiluted wine." Wine is mentioned throughout the Bible, from Noah's drunkenness to Jesus's first miracle at the wedding feast. From the decadence of Dionysus to the sublime celebration of the Christian Eucharist, wine encompasses the entire range of human experience. The Cretan author Kazantsakis, who was tormented by the tension between the carnal and the spiritual in his fiction and his own life, marveled at the capacity of wine to touch the very soul of man.

Though wine has accompanied man in his journey through civilization it has, until recently, been relatively and conspicuously absent from the American experience. American culture was first forged in the tradition of England and the northern European cultures, so beer and spirits have been the preferred alcoholic beverages. Wine was seen as the drink of a decadent aristocracy or those pretending to be part of such a class. Or it was associated with the hordes of impoverished, illiterate masses from southern Europe.

Today, Americans are rediscovering wine. Growth in red wine sales has been steep in the past decade, and red wine is shedding the unfortunate and undeserved prejudices previously associated with its consumption. And that's good. Because together with the olive, wine forms the foundation of a cuisine, and a lifestyle, that prolongs life and makes the added years that much more pleasurable. The Mediterraneans figured out the art of living long ago. By embracing the olive and the vine, we take tangible steps in our appreciation of that art.

Wine arouses passion. Therefore, it is not surprising that the debate over its benefits is sometimes passionate. After all, it seems paradoxical that promoters of health should advocate a substance that contains alcohol. Alcohol, like other mind-altering drugs, has been an accomplice to much human misery and violence. One only has to read Frank McCourt's *Angela's Ashes* or consider the

Alcohol and Blood Clotting

There is evidence that alcohol may help dissolve tiny blood clots once they form. You have probably heard of the new clot-busting drugs that doctors give people when they are having a heart attack. These drugs are based on the actions of tissue plasminogen activator (t-PA), which is kind of like Drano for a newly formed clot that is blocking coronary arteries. Despite contradictory evidence in a number of laboratory experiments, the Physicians Health Study showed that the level of t-PA is higher among alcohol consumers than abstainers and rises with the quantity of alcohol consumed on a regular basis.

carnage caused by drunk drivers to understand the spectrum of tragedy that alcohol abuse has caused. Yet the overwhelming majority of people who drink do so responsibly. And forcing those who do drink responsibly to abstain may actually increase their risk of death from heart disease. We should not casually advise people to consume a substance that is dangerous when misused. But we now know that alcohol, or at least red wine, can, through a variety of mechanisms, prevent heart disease. When we drink wine the way the French, Italians, or Greeks do, the potential for abuse is greatly reduced.

During the time I lived in Rome, only once did I see an Italian drunk, stumbling down the street. I vividly recall it because it was so unusual that it made an impression on me. Though many Italians drink wine every day, they consider it scandalous to be intoxicated. The Italian word for drunk is *umbriacone*, and it is a very shameful label.

The sobriety of Italians stood in stark contrast to the English-speaking subculture I knew in Rome. Many in this crowd seemed to live for Friday night, when they would go down to the Falcon Club near the Piazza Barberini and drink beer and hard liquor until they were practically unconscious or physically ill. Members of the English soccer team were notorious for coming to Rome, drinking beer until they were fall-down drunk, and starting fights.

Italians had a hard time understanding such barbarity and considered this behavior to be *schifoso*, or disgusting. They don't see alcohol primarily as an instrument of intoxication. Because they drink wine, they see it as a legitimate food replete with wonderful tastes and life-enhancing benefits. Of course, in the end the Italians, the French, the Spaniards, and the Portuguese will have the last laugh on the violent beer bingers with big bellies, because they will have outlived them.

The moral is, you should drink wine as the Italians—or the Greeks or the French—do. A little bit, every day, with food. These three guidelines—moderation, daily consumption, and consumption with food—are important to maximizing the benefits of wine, just as the dose, the frequency, and the manner of consumption are critical to maximizing a medicine's therapeutic benefits. Not only does this prescription sharply reduce the intoxicating effects of wine, but it is also vital to its health-promoting properties.

The argument for moderate drinking of red wine comes in two parts. First, there is a great deal of evidence that moderate alcohol consumption from any source—wine, beer, or liquor—is beneficial. Beyond that, there is also powerful evidence that red wine is especially beneficial.

The Evidence for Alcohol

When I was a student more than twenty years ago, a crusty old pathologist once told me, "Alcoholics always die with clean coronaries." By this he meant that his autopsies revealed that alcoholics almost never had clogged arteries, unlike most of the other autopsy cases. So although excessive drinking is deadly, it would not kill you through heart disease. This pathologist quoted no statistics or studies; it was just his personal experience over many years. As we shall see, the data have finally caught up with his observation.

Over the past decade there has been a great deal of study focused on the benefits of alcohol of all types. But this surge of interest was kicked off by wine, and of course by the French, who, as usual, were refusing to behave as the rest of the world expected. The French Paradox, a term coined by Dr. Serge Renaud, became famous when *60 Minutes* featured it on November 17, 1991. The paradox is simply this: When a large international research study, the MONICA (MONItoring CArdiovascular Disease) project, looked at diet and disease in twenty-seven different countries, researchers found that even though the French eat substantial amounts of saturated fat and smoke a great deal, they still have one of the lowest rates of heart disease in the world.

In an effort to explain this paradox, some researchers pointed out that the French consume enormous quantities of red wine. Could red wine protect against the otherwise harmful effects of saturated fat and smoking? After examining all the data, many came to the conclusion that it did.

Of course, other explanations were suggested along the way. For instance, as you head south in France, folks consume less saturated fat and more olive oil, and their mortality rate is lower than that of their countrymen in the north. In fact, the women in Toulouse in southern France are currently neck-and-neck with Japanese women for having the lowest heart disease rates and greatest longevity in the world. This is a statistical subtlety that gets lost in large national averages. The French are big cheese eaters, and others have suggested that saturated fat derived from cheese and other fermented dairy products like yogurt is somehow less harmful than that derived from meat. There is some evidence for this theory, but it remains controversial. And even when you take these other possibilities into account, it still seems that red wine does play an important role in preventing heart disease in France.

The medicinal qualities of wine have been recognized since the time of Homer. But the French Paradox and *60 Minutes* captured the imagination of the public and of researchers in a special way.

Since then, other large populations have been studied and old data have been reexamined, and virtually all have shown the same thing: Moderate alcohol consumption is heart healthy. The Copenhagen Heart Study followed 13,000 men and women for ten years and found that people who consumed one to two drinks a day had a 30 to 40 percent lower mortality rate. An American Cancer Society survey of 500,000 people found that those who consumed one to two drinks per day had a 20 percent lower overall mortality rate compared to non-drinkers. The famous Framingham Heart Study; the comprehensive Nurses' Health Study; a study of more than 100,000 Kaiser Permanente patients in California; and studies done in places as diverse as China, Scotland, Finland, Yugoslavia, and New Zealand all show similar results: One to two drinks a day protect against heart disease and death. These studies also consistently showed that after you exceed two

The Medicinal Value of Red Wine

This evidence must still be verified in humans, but recent experiments provide evidence that red wine has the biochemical
tools—phytochemicals—to do what the French Paradox and
other population studies suggest it can do: prevent disease.
(Almost all of these phytochemical compounds may also be
found in purple grape juice.) For instance, there are at least two
ways the phytochemicals in wine may inhibit platelet clotting,
thereby preventing heart attacks and strokes.

First, a substance in red wine, particularly American varieties, is salicylic acid—the active ingredient in aspirin. The reason
aspirin helps prevent heart disease is that the salicylic acid in
aspirin inhibits platelets from sticking together and forming blood
clots in coronary arteries. By drinking red wine daily, we are getting a small dose of aspirin every day. No wonder St. Paul
advised the disciple Timothy: *No longer drink only water, but take
a little wine for... your frequent ailments (Timothy 5:23.)* In other
words, take some aspirin and call me in the morning.

Second, certain other phytochemicals in grapes and red wine
such as resveratrol promote nitric oxide production. Nitric oxide
can also inhibit platelet clotting as well as help blood vessels
dilate. The benefits of nitric oxide have been understood only in
the past decade, but nitric oxide is now seen as an extremely
important player in preventing heart disease.

drinks a day, mortality starts going up and keeps going up as you
drink more.

The most frequent explanation for alcohol's ability to prevent
heart disease comes from the observation that alcohol can raise
levels of HDL, the good cholesterol. But some experts maintain
that this can account only for about 30 to 50 percent of the ben-

efit of alcohol. Recent evidence suggests that alcohol can also affect the proteins that sit on the surface of LDL cholesterol in a way that reduces risk. Other studies suggest that alcohol inhibits platelets from sticking together. Platelets are particles in your blood that rush to a site of injury and stick together to make your blood clot. Though this is important when you cut yourself, excessive clotting can clog up your coronary arteries.

Yet another way alcohol may protect against heart disease is through its effect on insulin. A recent study in the *British Medical Journal* suggests that alcohol can improve insulin sensitivity. Impaired insulin sensitivity, also called insulin resistance, is associated with higher insulin levels and a significantly increased risk of heart disease. By improving insulin sensitivity and raising HDL, alcohol may improve two features of the metabolic syndrome and reduce the risk of heart disease.

Alcohol, Stress, and Heart Disease

Stress reduction may also be a reason alcohol is heart healthy. While in my opinion wine eases the mind, lightens the soul, and relaxes the body in a special way, all forms of alcohol are used for stress reduction. Studying the effects of alcohol on stress and heart disease, however, is a little tricky. Are the stress-reducing properties of alcohol partly responsible for the reductions in heart disease? Or is it that more-relaxed, less-driven people are more likely to put away their briefcase for the evening and allow themselves a glass of wine? It's not clear. Certainly relying on alcohol to help you cope with life's problems is one of its most dangerous uses. Still I suspect that alcohol does play a role, however complicated, in reducing stress. And in this role I think wine has a unique niche. Because wine is a culturally based accompaniment to food rather than a specific tonic for stress reduction, like a martini, the deleterious effects of intentional self-medication with alcohol may be less for wine drinkers. Not fact, just opinion.

Alcohol: A Double-Edged Sword

That's the positive side of the story for alcohol. Are there any other concerns other than those related to alcoholism, pregnancy, drunk driving, and liver disease? Some population studies have suggested that alcohol may be related to breast cancer. After all, alcohol itself does have a pro-oxidant effect. But other studies such as the Framingham Heart Study have failed to show this association. And even in those studies that did show a relationship between alcohol and breast cancer it generally became significant only when women consumed more than a drink a day, with greater risks among premenopausal women. Moreover, these population studies often lump alcohol from all sources together, whether from vodka or red wine. French, Spanish, and Italian women have somewhat lower rates of breast cancer compared with Irish, English, and American women, even though the former group drinks considerably more alcohol, albeit in the form of red wine. After learning, as we soon will, about all the antioxidants in red wine that may have cancer-fighting potential, one could easily imagine why red wine might be very different from vodka in its effects on cancer and why red wine might even be protective. But this is speculation. Until we have better research many experts advise premenopausal women with a strong family history of breast cancer to avoid alcohol consumption. We concur, and suggest that high-risk women get their phytochemicals from purple grape juice, an excellent source, and save the red wine for special occasions.

For most people, however, the benefits of responsible alcohol consumption outweigh the risks. One demonstration of this comes from the researchers who analyzed the data from the Copenhagen Heart Study. These statisticians calculated that heavy drinking accounted for 117 deaths that could have been avoided by exercising moderation. On the other hand, they calculated that if everyone in the study had abstained from alcohol, there would have been 447 more deaths, mostly due to coronary heart disease. On balance, moderate consumption seems to do the greatest good for the greatest number.

Although such calculations are a bit contrived, they illustrate the point. The benefits of moderate drinking, as is done in Mediterranean countries, appear to outweigh the benefits of total abstinence for most people.

The Evidence for Red Wine

Alcohol in moderation, responsibly consumed, appears to be beneficial. But what about the frequent claims that red wine carries special advantages? That certainly is the message in the French Paradox. Is red wine indeed superior to beer, vodka, or even white wine, or is that merely a Mediterranean myth promulgated by the vendors of vino rosso?

It is not a myth. There is enough evidence available to demonstrate that red wine has special health-promoting properties.

First of all, red wine seems to have a greater effect on blood platelets than other alcoholic beverages do. Researcher Dr. John Folts of the University of Wisconsin found that red wine inhibits platelet clotting more than white wine or other types of alcohol do. It doesn't take much red wine to retard platelet clotting, but the effect lasts only twenty-four to forty-eight hours. This is one very important reason why daily consumption is so important and why weekend binge drinkers don't get this benefit. While there is evidence that alcohol alone can have this clot-inhibiting effect, Folts points out that it requires fairly high doses of alcohol, higher than what is achievable by moderate drinking. Fortunately, other substances in red wine enhance the platelet effect and enable you to achieve platelet inhibition at lower doses consistent with moderate consumption.

A bodybuilder friend once told me that it is customary to drink a little red wine before going onstage to compete. She insisted that red wine made the blood vessels dilate and appear more prominent—a definite plus for a competitive bodybuilder. At that time I dismissed the practice as bodybuilding folklore that was probably used to justify a little shot of courage before going onstage. But it turns out she was right: Red wine does dilate blood vessels. This is relevant to heart disease because red wine not only helps prevent the initial accumulation of cholesterol and platelet debris, but it also seems to help dilate coronary blood vessels to accommodate a greater flow of blood to the heart. Recent studies have related this to red wine's effect on nitric oxide as well as to its effect on prostacyclin. When Dr. Folts and other researchers such as Dr. Hashimoto from the University of Tokyo compared red wine with white wine and other forms of alcohol, they found that only red wine produced this artery-widening effect.

It seems that the most important contribution red wine makes to disease prevention is probably from its phytochemicals. Nature puts extra doses of phytochemicals in deeply colored fruits and vegetables. So it should not be surprising that red wine has an unusually generous supply of these life-preserving compounds.

Beer and white wine both have some phytochemicals, but red wine has far more. Spirits have virtually none.

Most of the phytochemicals in red wine are in a class called flavonoids, which are part of a larger group called polyphenols. Flavonoids play an important role in preventing the oxidation of LDL cholesterol. As you know, the level of oxidized LDL is one of the strongest predictors of heart disease because oxidized LDL is the angry biologic agent that gets the artery wrecking ball rolling. Prevent LDL from oxidizing, and you go a long way toward preventing heart disease. Some of these phytochemicals also seem to play a role in suppressing inflammation and in inhibiting the creation and propagation of cancer cells.

Dr. Folts argues that these phytochemicals are more important than alcohol for explaining wine's benefits. His research shows that it is the phytochemicals in red wine that inhibit platelet clotting and cause blood vessels to dilate. As evidence he points to white wine's anemic and often nonexistent effects on platelet clotting and blood vessel dilation, particularly at doses consistent with moderate drinking. Furthermore, he has shown that purple grape juice also can inhibit platelets from sticking together and cause blood vessels to dilate. There is even evidence to show that grape juice can lower LDL cholesterol. This is because even though grape juice is devoid of alcohol, it contains virtually all the phytochemicals that red wine does. Purple grape juice provides a reasonable alternative for people who cannot or prefer not to drink alcohol or red wine. Unfortunately grape juice will never complement a plate of pasta puttanesca or pan-seared trout like a nice pinot noir. (Yes, you can have red wine with fish.)

Still one more way in which phytochemicals in red wine may prevent heart disease was demonstrated by Drs. Katsuya Iijima and Masayoshi Hashimoto in Japan. It seems that when coronary blood vessels are damaged by cholesterol, they often grow more of the tiny smooth muscle cells that are normally in the walls of the coronary arteries. Unfortunately, these new muscles only make matters worse because they further thicken the wall of the blood vessel and further impede the flow of blood to the heart. These researchers found that phytochemicals from red wine inhibited the unwanted growth of these tiny muscle fibers in the arteries of rats. Does this mean that wine has the same effect in humans? We don't know, but it's certainly a possibility that deserves further research.

It is not surprising that my Italian immigrant grandfather, who made and drank his own wine, was an advocate of vino rosso. But he drank it because it was his cultural inheritance. Surprisingly, it was my Irish immigrant grandfather who was the staunchest advocate of the medicinal value of red wine. Every morning he would rise at four o'clock and say his prayers. Then he would head to the kitchen for his usual daily breakfast: two raw eggs mixed in a glass of port wine. He would down his health cocktail like a Hibernian Rocky Balboa in training and then head out to work. Despite the protests of his daughters, he insisted that this was a healthy breakfast and gave him the strength he needed at work. Pop, as we called him, lived to an alert and vigorous ninety.

The olive and the fruit of the vine complement each other not only in taste but in health. These two biblical foods form the foundation of Mediterranean cuisine and are the elixirs of health in that part of the world. If we consume them wisely, they can do the same for us.

Red Wine's Health-Enhancing Substances

Although much of the following information is from test tubes and animals, it is interesting to think that these substances may contribute to health in humans.

Anthocyanin. A flavonoid that provides the red pigment in grapes. As an antioxidant, anthocyanin not only stops LDL from dangerously being oxidized, it has also been shown to inhibit an enzyme that causes cholesterol production. In addition, anthocyanin has been shown to prevent blood clots.

Caffeic acid. An antioxidant with antibacterial and anticarcinogenic effects. Also found in olive oil (see page 160).

Catechin. This flavonoid has been shown to reduce bad cholesterol oxidation and decrease blood clotting in arteries. It also preserves alpha tocopherol (vitamin E) and beta carotene in the body. In laboratory rats, it has been shown to reduce blood glucose levels and may thereby have a beneficial effect on insulin.

Cinnamic acid. A polyphenol that has been shown to inhibit the growth of cancer cells. The salicylic acid in red wine is manufactured from cinnamic acid.

Ellagic acid. Neutralizes potential carcinogens, rendering them incapable of attacking DNA, and prevents oxidized LDL from damaging cells.

Epicatechin. Enhances an antioxidant enzyme that inhibits blood lipid oxidation.

Ferulic acid An antioxidant and an anticarcinogenic acid. Also found in olive oil (see page 161).

Fisetin. A flavonoid that inhibits the oxidation of LDL and helps preserve the vitamin E content of the LDL cholesterol particle. It discourages inflammation and the clotting of blood platelets in animals by inhibiting the effects of thromboxane, an evil prostaglandin. It has also been shown to stop the growth of cancer cells in a laboratory test tube.

Gentisic acid. A metabolite or breakdown product of salicylic acid, the aspirin-like compound found in red wines. Gentisic acid is an antioxidant and an anti-inflamatory but also seems to have very potent antibacterial properties. According to Dr. Carlos Muller, a professor of enology at California State University at Fresno, American grapes are bred to be more infection-resistant than many European varieties. That is why you will find more salicylic acid and gentisic acid in American varieties of red wine. In fact, in certain European reds it can be hard to find any salicylic acid, and hence its metabolites such as gentisic acid, at all.

Leucocyanidol. Leucocyanidol, by its effect on certain prostaglandins, may play a role in inhibiting the inflammation of blood vessels associated with coronary artery disease. It can also induce relaxation and dilatation in rat blood vessels by enhancing the synthesis of nitric oxide. As an antioxidant this versatile compound is a potent scavenger of free radicals.

P-coumaric. Another polyphenol, P-coumaric helps prevent the formation of potentially carcinogenic nitrosamines formed during digestion of processed meats.

Polydatin. Shown, in a test tube, to inhibit platelet aggregation and therefore clotting.

Quercetin. Quercetin is an antioxidant. It also discourages clotting, promotes dilatation of blood vessels, and discourages inflammation. In a test tube it inhibits the growth of cancer cells.

Resveratrol. Another flavonoid, resveratrol has been shown to stop LDL oxidation. It also promotes blood vessel dilatation and reduces platelet stickiness through two possible mechanisms. First, it enhances nitric oxide production. Second, it promotes prostacyclin while suppressing thromboxane. Resveratrol maximizes prostacyclin and minimizes thromboxane by inhibiting an enzyme called cyclooxengenase II (COX II). In the right doses COX II inhibitors have also been shown to prevent certain kinds of cancer, especially colon cancer. In addition, they reduce the pain and inflammation associated with arthritis.

Salicylic acid. Closely related to acetylsalicylic acid or aspirin, salicylic acid shares most of the same properties as aspirin, which, despite its long history, is turning out to be one of the miracle compounds of the decade. Also a cyclooxygenase or COX inhibitor, aspirin (and salicylic acid) has a multitude of effects but is most famous for its ability to suppress inflammation and to prevent platelets from sticking together, which in turn prevents blood from clotting and clogging up coronary arteries. The regular use of aspirin is associated with decreased risk of heart disease, stroke, and colon cancer in humans. Eight ounces of wine contain about 5 milligrams of salicylic acid. In wine, salicylic acid is made from cinnamic acid. As stated, some experts feel that some American grapes are likely to have more salicylic acid than many European grapes and wines do.

Tannic acid. A polyphenol tannic acid has been shown in a test tube to promote dilation of blood vessel tissue from rats through its effect on nitric oxide. Tannins have been shown to reduce the activity of a number of carcinogens and to function as antioxidants.

Taxifolin Another flavonoid, taxifolin has been shown in a test tube to inhibit lipid oxidation.

Vanillic acid. Antibacterial, antifungal.

Part Three:
Applying the Mediterranean Diet to Your Life

15
Seven Characteristics of an Effective Diet

The way of eating and living we are about to show you is not meant to be a rigid "diet" in the way most of us usually use that term. It's a way of life. And for life you need more than rules; you need understanding. That's what we tried to give you in the preceding chapters.

Of course, there will be a few rules in the pages to come—especially while you are still in the losing weight phase. No matter what other diet books tell you, you can't actually lose weight without cutting calories, or adding exercise while keeping calories the same, or doing both (the best way). So in the following chapters we do give you some meal plans that are limited to a certain number of calories, as well as a Mediterranean approach to exercise. The good news is, the food in these meal plans is so good and filling that it should be easy to stick to the limits.

We will start by explaining what we believe are the key ingredients of a successful diet. We call them the seven characteristics of an effective diet. Knowing these basic principles should help you better understand the meal plans and recipes and adapt them to your own life.

Earlier we noted that diet can be defined in two ways. One definition is "a temporary intervention to lose weight." Most Americans seem to go on and off such diets all the time, because these diets rarely work in the long term. The other definition is "simply a way to eat *as part of a fully integrated lifestyle.*" The word "diet" in Italy, Tunisia, and Greece describes how people in a certain culture eat. These diets are not interventionist or adopted for a specific objective. They are an end in themselves. And, of course, some are healthier or more palatable than others. Yet one advantage they all have is that they establish natural guidelines, even instincts, for eating; rules that have evolved over hundreds or thousands of years and are reinforced by culture, family, and friends—all of whom eat the same way. People stick to such a diet because it is woven into the fabric of their lives.

We Americans do not have that advantage. Most of us have long since left behind the cultural diet of our immigrant forebears and adopted the unhealthy American diet, which lacks the boundaries and guidelines of older, culturally based cuisines. Dominated by convenience, quantity, and continual consumption, the American diet is dangerous.

But there is a bright side: Because Americans are not tied to a culturally restrictive way of eating, they are free to choose alternatives. The Mediterranean diet offers one of the best alternatives, because it embodies all the characteristics of an effective diet. It is suitable not only for everyday living, but for health and weight loss. Moreover, this diet is familiar to most of us. And remember, though we may consciously adopt it as a diet in the first sense, it is also a way of eating that is meant to last a lifetime.

Here are the seven characteristics of an effective diet:

1. simplicity

2. palatability and diversity

3. satiety

4. durability

5. universality

6. nutritional value

7. harmony

1. Simplicity. Most of us are not gourmet chefs and cannot tackle complicated recipes. Besides, who has the time to buy exotic ingredients, learn new dishes, and take the time to cook them? By "simplicity" we mean food that is easy and quick to prepare. If you ask people why past diets failed, a frequent response is, "Not enough time [to prepare the food, eat the food, and follow the rules]." Mediterranean cooking is one of the simplest cuisines in the world to master. The essential ingredients, which can be combined in a variety of ways, are so mutually compatible that it is almost impossible to make a mistake. And because quick sauces are central to the cuisine, preparation time is short and leftovers can be easily reheated. Many of the recipes can be prepared in large batches and frozen for future use. We make it even simpler by providing you with a basic list of foods to keep on hand (see page 200). With this list, you will always have the foods and ingredients necessary to make a delicious meal.

2. Palatability and Diversity. A diet must be tasty if you expect to follow it for the long term. It's hard to say whether it's worse to be on a diet that leaves you hungry or one that doesn't taste good, both of which characterize most low-fat diets. Not so of the true Mediterranean diet, which may be the most flavorful diet in the world.

A big part of palatability is diversity. Even if something tastes good, eating it every day will eventually bore you. Boredom will never be a problem with the Mediterranean diet, which is blessed with enormous diversity. Italian cooking alone has a multitude of wonderful dishes, to which we can add Greek, Spanish, and many French, Middle Eastern, and even North African dishes.

3. Satiety. Satiety—feeling full, not hungry—is obviously critical to the success of a diet. People won't stay on a diet that leaves them hungry. Fats and carbohydrates both contribute to satiety. Carbohydrate-rich food, especially fiber-rich carbohydrates like vegetables, can create physical distension of the stomach and an immediate sense of fullness. But you will probably get hungry again quickly—within an hour or two. Dietary fat, on the other hand, sends special messages to the brain that give you a sense of satiety and delay the time until you feel hungry again. Protein does the same. So, satisfaction requires a well-balanced mix of protein, carbohydrate, and fat, plus a good dose of fiber—exactly what you find in the Mediterranean diet.

4. Durability. Durability is the track record of a diet in the real world. Diets that have been durable over centuries have evolved slowly and been perfected. They offer a level of consistency and confidence that fad diets just can't reach. The Mediterranean diet is one of the oldest and most stable diets in Western civilization.

And after all these centuries, modern science has proved it to be one of the healthiest diets in the world.

5. *Universality.* No diet appeals to everyone, but some have broader appeal than others. Broad appeal is essential, because food is part of fellowship. Choosing a diet that few others find appetizing creates barriers to fellowship and practical problems for families. The Mediterranean diet is one of the most universally accepted cuisines. You can find Italian restaurants from Sicily to Dublin and from Seattle to Miami. True, some people don't like capers and others don't like mushrooms or broccoli, but there are enough diverse ingredients to suit any taste. Even those who think they dislike olive oil will usually enjoy the small amount we recommend blended with the other flavors in the foods and spices (or they can use the relatively taste-free canola oil).

Most of the ingredients, moreover, are available all over the world—and are as close as your local supermarket. Exotic, hard-to-find ingredients are just one more barrier that can knock you off your diet.

6. *Nutritional Value.* As we now know, the Mediterranean diet documented by Ancel Keys in the Seven Country Study is associated with remarkably lower rates of chronic disease and premature death. A nutritious diet doesn't just cover the minimum daily requirements of vitamins, minerals, protein, and calories. A nutritious diet fights the diseases of modern life such as heart maladies, diabetes, cancer, and hypertension; it also boosts health by incorporating as many phytochemicals and micronutrients as possible. A good diet also minimizes saturated fats, easily oxidizes polyunsaturated fats, and *eliminates* the risks of synthetic compounds like trans fats and Olestra.

In a country suffering from an epidemic of obesity, a nutritious diet can be easily adapted to weight loss without bizarre changes. You don't change how you cook or shop, you just measure a little more carefully and eat a little less, which will be easy to do because your food will still be delicious and filling.

7. Harmony. Harmony is not something most of us naturally associate with diets—especially fad diets. But in some ways harmony is the most important ingredient. Harmony enables a diet to become a way of life, a daily routine. The opposite of harmony is conflict—with our lifestyle, our tastes, our families, our bodies, or even among the ingredients themselves.

Harmony among the elements of a diet is essential to its nutritional and culinary success. The harmony in the Mediterranean diet is astounding on all these different levels. Basil, tomatoes, garlic, and olive oil complement each other so perfectly that one might think God had the combination in mind when he created these foods. As if that weren't enough, this seductive but simple combination supplies such a remarkable spectrum of health-promoting nutrients that it again seems as if divine intervention played a role. And there is still more: Broccoli, spinach, potatoes, pasta, bread, pine nuts, oregano, cannellini beans, mozzarella, wine, capers, olives, fish, and meat in sensible, flavorful proportions, as well as delicious fruits, nuts, and vegetables, can all be added to the basic combination or to each other in endless permutations. And somehow they always combine to create a satisfying, highly palatable meal.

This diet has visual harmony as well. It has been said that we eat first with our eyes. The varied and harmonious colors and textures in a typical Mediterranean recipe are such that even the simplest recipe presents an appetizing picture.

Harmony has practical implications because it contributes to simplicity. Because the basic couple of dozen ingredients harmonize so well, you need keep only a limited food inventory on hand. Recipes build on one another, as do cooking techniques, therefore simplifying shopping, meal planning, and preparation. You can easily master the basic food combinations and develop an intimate knowledge of the elements from the perspective of taste, preparation, and nutrition. With a limited number of things to remember it won't be long before you know that a cup of pasta has about two hundred calories, a cup of spinach or broccoli about fifty calories, and a teaspoon of olive oil forty calories—or before you make up your own recipes because you are in tune with the unifying harmonies of the diet.

16
Making the Healthiest Diet Your Diet

In the following pages we provide you with everything you need to start eating and living healthfully on the Mediterranean diet. We have included recipes and recipe hints and a list of basic items you should keep on hand.

The Mediterranean diet involves a variety of foods. But you don't have to count every single calorie or figure out fat grams and percentages. There is only one thing you need to account for—portion size—and only three things you should measure at first—olive oil; starches, especially pasta; and meat (which is not a big part of the diet anyway). But you will eventually be able to tell by sight how much of an item you have. When first incorporating Mediterranean foods into your life, figure out how many teaspoons of oil it takes to fill the cap of the olive oil bottle so you can use it to measure, or notice how two teaspoons of olive oil look in the pan. At first, weigh long pasta and measure short pasta by the cup (before cooking). Meat is usually easy. Three ounces of meat is about the size of a deck of cards. Try to use the same size plate so you can begin to tell how much space the desired amount of pasta/rice/potato meat occupies. You will soon know what the size of a cooked portion looks like, even when eating out. But, in the beginning, measure the oil, starches, and meat. Remember, it is your *overall* caloric intake that determines weight loss or weight gain, and these foods can add calories quickly if you don't pay attention. Fruits and nonstarchy vegetables like spinach and broccoli can be eaten in almost unlimited amounts.

- Short pastas like ziti are approximately 200 calories per cup dry weight.

- Long pasta like linguini or spaghetti must be weighed on a scale; 2 ounces equal 200 calories.

- Olive oil is 120 calories per tablespoon and 40 calories per teaspoon.

You Are What You Buy

Aristotle, the great philosopher, was Greek, so we know he ate a Mediterranean diet. One of Aristotle's great contributions to philosophy was the syllogism, a series of statements so constructed that if you accept the first premise you have to accept the conclusion. We suspect that at some point he must have deduced the following syllogism as he watched Athenians buying food in the *Agora*, the square that contained the open-air markets:

> If you are what you eat,
> And you eat what you buy,
> Then you are what you buy.

If it's not in the house, not visible, or out of reach, you won't eat it. So the first step in an effective diet is to keep the right stuff in your house and the wrong stuff out. Get rid of all the junk in your cupboards and refrigerator and banish fast food from your life.

You are what you buy. You must stop buying sweets, chips, hamburger meat, and highly processed foods like Snackwells and no-fat salad dressing. If they're in your house, throw them out—*today*. You need about fifty food items in your house at all times if you want to eat healthfully and control or lose weight on a healthy Mediterranean diet (see page 200 for list).

> Buy plenty of frozen vegetables, especially green vegetables, which are key to weight loss and health. You can't eat too much of them.

And the Mediterranean diet is not expensive. In fact, because of its peasant origins, it is downright cheap—no special weight-loss foods and products as with some other diets.

You should try to get to the store at least once a week to restock fresh items. But if you are working sixty hours a week it can be hard. Have enough staples on hand so you can throw a dinner together even if you haven't shopped for two weeks. If you stock up on canned, jarred, and frozen items you may not have to restock those items for months, making the weekly trips for fresh foods a lot quicker. A big reason people fail on diets is that when they look for something to eat they never have the right things, and have too much of the wrong things. A well-stocked inventory is the secret to success. You can add other Mediterranean-friendly items to the list, but this list covers the basics.

And remember, every time you do go to the store, get more fresh fruit and vegetables. You can't have too many. The minimum is three pieces of fruit a day—that means buying at least twenty-one pieces of fruit a week. Keep a supply of fresh fruit at work.

There may be some things in the Mediterranean diet you think you don't like, such as anchovies or capers. Don't worry, they are just minor ingredients. As part of the overall harmony of the diet they will blend in beautifully with the other ingredients. You might never have known they were there if you hadn't cooked them yourself. Of course, if you don't want to use them, you don't have to.

Lots of items on the list are dried, canned, or jarred. Be efficient and stock up. They will last a long time and always be on hand. And remember, canned and frozen fruits and vegetables are very nutritious. So even if you can't get to the store to buy the fresh produce, you will always be able to make a good meal with what you have in the house.

Fifty Basics to Have in Stock

The items on this list are all you need to make the recipes for the Mediterranean weight-loss program (see page 229).

1. anchovy fillets or paste

2. artichokes—canned or jarred

3. asparagus—canned or frozen

4. beans—canned (such as cannellini, red beans, and chickpeas)

5. bread—pita or high-fiber

6. breakfast cereal—especially high fiber, minimum 5 grams fiber per serving (such as Shredded Wheat, oatmeal, Fiber One, Grape Nuts, and All Bran)

7. broccoli—frozen

8. canola oil

9. capers

10. carrots—fresh

11. cheese—like swiss, provolone(nothing wrong with an occasional piece, but don't overdo it—you want to stay away from saturated fat), also grated parmesan or romano, part-skim mozzarella

12. chicken/beef broth—canned or bouillon cubes

13. chicken breasts

14. clams—canned

15. eggs

16. feta cheese—crumbled

17. fruits—canned (such as peaches and pears packed in juice, not syrup)

18. garlic cloves

19. grape juice—purple (especially if you can't drink alcohol or red wine)

20. green/red peppers—fresh

21. ham—lean and sliced (use only occasionally)

22. herbs and spices (such as salt, red pepper flakes, black pepper, fresh or dried basil, oregano, parsley, and rosemary)

23. lemons—fresh

24. lentils—dry

25. lentil soup—canned

26. milk—nonfat

27. mushrooms—fresh and canned

28. olive oil—preferably extra virgin

29. olives—canned and packed in brine (sliced, whole)

30. onions—red and white

31. pasta—short noodles like ziti for easy measuring, preferably high-fiber, 4 grams of fiber per serving (for good tasting, high-fiber pasta try Delverde whole-wheat pasta)

32. peas—canned or frozen

33. pine nuts (pignolis)

34. potatoes—fresh

35. raisins

36. red wine—one half-glass to one glass with dinner (omit if there is a health reason preventing you from drinking wine)

37. rice—preferably brown (brown rice is higher in fiber and more nutritious)

38. roasted red peppers—jarred

39. shrimp—frozen

40. spinach/kale—frozen

41. tomatoes—canned and paste

42. tomatoes—fresh (in season)

43. tuna—canned in water

44. turkey—sliced (occasional use of meat is okay, but avoid ground beef)

45. various fresh fruits in season (such as grapes, figs, tangerines, plums, oranges, strawberries, apples, etc.)—three times a day

46. various fresh vegetables in season (such as arugula eggplant, spinach, broccoli, broccoli rabe, kale, asparagus, cucumbers, etc.)

47. vegetable medleys—frozen

48. vinegar—balsamic

49. walnuts and other nuts—shelled

50. yogurt—plain

Recipes for Nutrition and Weight Loss

The recipes in this section were designed by Dr. Mary Flynn for a Mediterranean diet weight-loss program at Brown University. They were reviewed by chef Mary Melie at Christopher Martins restaurant in New Haven, Connecticut. Most of the recipes were also tested in our Mediterranean diet weight-loss group. All the recipes can be made with ingredients from the above "fifty basics" food list, and are integrated with the weight-loss meal plans on page 229. All these recipies were designed with weight loss, simplicity, and time in mind—virtually all can be prepared by the novice cook in less than twenty minutes. These recipes are meant as a general guide to get you to start cooking simply and nutritiously. Experiment freely with the procedures and the ingredients. You can substitute vegetables and herbs, depending on what you have available, what you like, or what is in season. One of the great things about Mediterranean cooking is its simple preparation. It is almost impossible to produce something inedible.

Breakfast

Many Mediterraneans eat light "continental" breakfasts; they may have fruit, yogurt, or fiber-rich bread with fruit spread (eggs, occasionally). Many Americans are accustomed to eating cereal for breakfast, so we have listed some of the healthier, high-fiber cereals below. Bland cereals come to life when berries or other fruit are added—remember, you can't have too much fruit.

Never skip breakfast. By eating a good breakfast (250 to 400 calories) every morning you will better control your caloric intake for the rest of the day. From the selections below, pick two or three that you like and stick with them and adjust portions and calories according to your personal needs (see meal plans on page 229 for recommended calorie intakes).

- High-fiber cereals: Fiber One, All Bran, Bran Buds
    1 cup of cereal with 1/2 cup of skim milk = about 150 calories—add fruit or berries

- Hot cereals: Oatmeal (regular/quick/instant), Cream of Wheat—use plain or unsweetened variety and add nuts, raisins, or fruit
    150 to 250 calories per cup

- Soft boiled egg (one or two) with one slice of whole wheat bread (eating eggs by themselves does not raise blood cholesterol; frying them in butter or bacon fat does)
    155 calories (1 egg = 80 calories; 1 slice of wheat bread = 75 calories)

- Plain yogurt (regular, low-fat, or nonfat without added sugar) with fresh fruit
    150 to 250 calories

- Two thick slices of high-fiber, fresh whole wheat bread with low-sugar fruit spread
    about 300 calories

- Granola with yogurt (below is a recipe for granola made with olive oil that is easy and delicious)
    350 to 450 calories

Granola

8 servings—240 calories per serving

    2 cups regular rolled oats
    1/2 cup slivered almonds
    1/2 cup honey
    1/3 cup olive oil
    1/2 cup raisins

Preheat oven to 300 degrees. In a large bowl mix oats and almonds. Make a well in the mixture, pour in the honey and oil, and mix together. The mixture will be sticky but should stir together. Spread the mixture in a 15x10x1" baking pan and bake for 15 minutes. Stir mixture in pan and bake for an additional 10 to 15 minutes or until mixture is golden brown (check every 5 minutes to prevent burning).

Lunch and Side Dishes

Try to bring your lunch to work (have plenty of tupperware on hand). You can use some of the leftovers from your Mediterranean dinners, or prepare lunch as you are cleaning up from dinner the night before. If you buy your lunch look for soups, salads, and meatless dishes. Be conscious of your portion sizes, and be careful with sandwiches. White bread, rolls, and crackers are the biggest source of calories in the American diet (donuts, cookies, and cakes are number two—stay away). Try eating half a sandwich instead of a whole one, and try using pita bread to reduce your daily caloric intake. Instead of the usual high-in-saturated-fat condiments like mayonnaise, use a dash of olive oil–based dressing or a little mustard on your sandwich. Don't forget to pick up a piece of fruit for your Mediterranean snack.

Basic Olive Oil Dressing

12 servings—80 calories per serving

> 1/4 cup vinegar
> 3/4 cup olive oil
> dash of seasonings to taste (basil, oregano, garlic powder, pepper, salt, etc.)

Whisk the above ingredients together in a small bowl. Store in a covered container and refrigerate until ready to use.

Cheese and Roasted Red Pepper Sandwich

1 serving—340 calories per serving

> 1 ounce cheese, such as feta, mozzarella, provolone, or Swiss
> 2 to 4 roasted red pepper slices, jarred or homemade

1 tablespoon olive oil dressing (see page 204)

leafy greens like romaine, arugula, or any dark green
   lettuce

2 slices whole-wheat bread

Pile cheese, peppers, dressing, and greens on one slice of bread
and top with the other slice.

Option: Substitute tomato slices for red peppers.

Italian Pasta Salad

2 servings—540 calories per serving

6 ounces cooked pasta

6 tablespoons olive oil dressing (see page 204)

Various chopped greens and vegetables (red and green
   peppers, tomatoes, cucumbers, carrots, etc.)

Mix together above ingredients in medium bowl and serve.

Italian Potato Salad

2 servings—380 calories per serving

2 cups potato, boiled and cubed

6 tablespoons olive oil dressing (see page 204)

Various chopped greens and vegetables (red and green
   peppers, tomatoes, cucumbers, carrots, etc.)

Mix all ingredients in a medium bowl and serve.

Italian Tuna Salad

2 servings—350 calories per serving

1 6-ounce can tuna packed in water

6 tablespoons olive oil dressing (see page 204)
Various chopped greens and vegetables red and green
peppers, tomatoes, cucumbers, carrots, etc.)

Mix all ingredients in a medium bowl and serve on lettuce leaves
or in sandwiches.

Mediterranean Baked Potato

*An average 5-inch baking potato is about 220 calories before adding
olive oil.*

1 serving—260–340 calories per serving

1 baking potato, washed and pierced several times
with fork
1 teaspoon to 1 tablespoon olive oil
salt and pepper to taste

Preheat the oven to 450 degrees. Bake the potato for one hour or
until the potato is soft (test by piercing with fork). Remove from
oven, split in half, and add the olive oil, and salt and pepper to
taste.

Mediterranean Bean Salad

2 servings—390 calories per serving

1 1/2 cups garbanzo beans (chickpeas) or cannellini
beans, drained and rinsed
4 tablespoons olive oil dressing (see page 204)
Various chopped greens and vegetables (red and green
peppers, tomatoes, cucumbers, carrots, etc.)

Mix all ingredients in a medium bowl and serve.

Mediterranean Rice _____

Brown rice is healthier for you but takes a little longer to make, about 40 minutes. One cup of dry rice yields 2 cups cooked and adds up to about 400 calories without the oil.
2 servings—240 calories per serving

>   2 cups water
>   1/2 teaspoon salt
>   1 cup rice
>   2 teaspoons olive oil

Bring the water and salt to a boil in a medium pot. Add the rice and the oil. Reduce heat to medium low, cover, and cook for 17 to 20 minutes, or until all the water is absorbed.

Mediterranean Sandwich _____

1 serving—300 calories per serving

>   1 ounce fresh mozzarella
>   3 to 4 spinach leaves
>   1 whole roasted red pepper, jarred or homemade
>   2 marinated artichokes, jarred
>   1 tablespoon olive oil or olive oil dressing (see page
>   204)
>   1 pita

Place mozzarella, spinach, pepper, artichokes, and oil or dressing in pita and enjoy.

Peppers, Mushrooms, and Onion Pocket _____

Feel free to add or substitute eggplant, broccoli, or any other colorful vegetable in this recipe.

1 serving—300 calories per serving

> 1 tablespoon olive oil
> 1 garlic clove, peeled and minced
> 1 green pepper, diced
> 1 red pepper, diced
> 1/4 cup onion, diced
> 1/4 cup mushrooms, diced
> fresh or dried herbs, suchas basil, oregano, or rose-
> > mary
> 1 medium pita pocket

Heat the oil in a skillet over medium high heat. Add the garlic and cook for 2 to 3 minutes. Add the peppers, onion, mushrooms, and herbs and stir to coat with the oil. Cook for 5 to 8 minutes, stirring often. Stuff vegetable mixture into a pita pocket and enjoy.

Note: Make extra vegetable mixture to serve as a side dish for dinner with chicken or fish.

Roasted or Grilled Vegetables _____

Roasted or grilled vegetables are very versatile. You can use them as a warm or cold side dish, in a pita pocket sandwich, or tossed with pasta for a warm or cold pasta meal.

6 1/2-cup servings—75 calories per serving

> 1 red pepper, seeded and diced
> 1 green pepper, seeded and diced
> 1 small eggplant, diced (with or without peel)

1 onion, diced

whole, peeled garlic cloves to taste

1/3 cup olive oil

salt and pepper to taste

Preheat oven to 400 degrees. Place peppers, eggplant, onions, and garlic in a roasting pan. Drizzle olive oil over vegetables and season with salt (salt lightly or vegetable liquid will run) and pepper to taste. Roast vegetables in oven, stirring every 10 to 15 minutes, for 40 minutes or until desired doneness.

Grilled: Use the same ingredients but omit garlic and cut the vegetables into 2-inch strips. Brush vegetables with olive oil and place on a preheated grill. Cook until desired tenderness, turning frequently.

Spinach Pocket

This is a great, tasty, filling lunch that is loaded with phytochemicals. Make extra and freeze for future lunches.
2 servings—300 calories per serving

2 tablespoons olive oil

1 garlic clove, peeled and minced

1 10-ounce package of frozen, chopped spinach
   (defrosted and drained)

fresh or dried herbs like basil, oregano, or rosemary
   to taste

1 medium pita pocket

Heat the oil in a skillet over medium high heat. Add the garlic and cook for 2 to 3 minutes. Add the spinach, stir to coat with oil, and heat through, about 3 to 4 minutes. Stir in the herbs. Stuff the spinach mixture into a pita pocket.

Options: Use frozen, chopped broccoli instead of spinach; sprinkle with grated cheese before serving; or add a dash of hot red pepper flakes to the oil and garlic.

Mediterranean Mashed Potatoes _____

2 servings—200 calories per serving

> 2 cups boiled potatoes
> 2 tablespoons olive oil
> 4 tablespoons nonfat milk
> salt and pepper to taste

Using a fork or potato masher, mix all ingredients together in a medium bowl. Add salt and pepper to taste and serve with chicken or fish.

Strawberry Spinach Salad _____

6 servings—215 calories per serving

> 1 pound bag frozen strawberries, defrosted and juices
>   reserved
> 1/4 cup olive oil (not extra virgin)
> 1/3 cup white vinegar
> 1 tablespoon sugar
> 1/2 teaspoon salt
> 1 clove garlic
> dash pepper
> 1 pound bag fresh spinach, washed

Combine all ingredients except spinach in a medium bowl and marinate at least 1 hour (up to 8 hours). Place the spinach in a large bowl and pour strawberry dressing on top. Toss and serve.

Soups

Soups are relatively easy to prepare. They can be simmered slowly for a more robust flavor, but you can eat them as soon as the ingredients are heated through. Soups can also be made in quantity and frozen in large containers or in individual serving sizes. If you make soup to freeze and use later, you might consider doing so without the pasta, rice, or potato components. These starch items do not freeze as well as the rest of the soup. You can add them when you're ready to reheat the soup. Soups can, of course, be used for lunch as well as dinner.

Broccoli Soup

5 servings—57 calories per serving

> 1 pound fresh broccoli, heads and tender stems chopped
> 5 cups chicken stock
> salt and pepper to taste
> 1 tablespoon lemon juice

Bring the stock to a boil in a large pot over medium heat. Add the broccoli and simmer until soft, about 30 minutes. Purée the soup in a food processor or blender, return to pot, add lemon juice, salt, and pepper.

Note: For a heartier soup, add a 1/2 cup cooked pasta or rice after soup is puréed.

Escarole and Bean Soup

6 servings—310 calories per serving

> 3 tablespoons extra-virgin olive oil

Ways to Use Olive Oil

Vegetables:

- add to cooked or raw vegetables.

- coat any vegetable with olive oil and roast it. You can roast in a preheated 400 degree oven. The roasting time will vary depending on the types of vegetables and how soft you want them. Most are done in 15 to 20 minutes. But make sure you check them as they cook.

Roasted vegetables can be eaten hot, as is, or tossed with pasta. You can also cool them and use them in a pasta or tortellini salad (use olive oil dressing).

- brush olive oil on vegetables and cook on a grill. Keep an eye on them, as they can cook fast.

Fish:

lean white fish (about 30 calories per ounce): sea bass, cod, flounder, grouper, haddock, perch, pollack, orange roughy, skip-jack tuna

medium fat fish (35-40 calories per ounce): freshwater bass, snapper, canned tuna, coho salmon

higher fat fish (50-60 calories per ounce): Florida pampano, halibut, Atlantic salmon, chinook salmon, trout

- put the olive oil on any fish and bake or grill. You can add fresh or dried herbs to the oil for a variety of flavors.

2 cloves garlic

3 to 4 cups escarole, cut into bite-sized pieces

7 cups chicken broth

1 19-ounce can cannellini beans, rinsed and drained

8 ounces cooked pasta

Heat the oil in a large soup pot over medium heat. Lower the heat to medium low and stir in the garlic and escarole. Cook for about 5 minutes or until the escarole is wilted. Add the beans, broth, and cooked pasta. Stir to combine and heat through, about 5 minutes and serve.

Lentil Soup

8 servings—215 calories per serving

3 tablespoons olive oil

1/4 pound lean cooked ham, cut into small cubes (optional)

3 garlic cloves, peeled and chopped

1 medium onion, peeled and chopped

2 carrots, trimmed and thinly sliced

7 cups chicken broth

1 1/2 cups dry lentils

sprig of lemon thyme

2 to 3 bay leaves

Heat 1 tablespoon olive oil in large soup pot over medium heat. Add ham and cook about 5 minutes. Remove meat and set aside. Add the remaining oil, garlic, onion, and carrots and reduce heat to low. Cover and cook for about 25 minutes. Add chicken broth, lentils, thyme, and bay leaves. Raise heat to medium high and bring to a boil. Lower heat, cover, and cook for 45 minutes. Remove thyme and bay leaves. Return ham to pot and heat 2 minutes.

Note: Make plenty of lentil soup to freeze and use for future lunches and dinners.

Tomato and Clam Soup

6 servings—300 calories per serving

> 3 tablespoons extra-virgin olive oil
>
> 1 medium onion, peeled and chopped
>
> 2 cloves garlic, peeled and chopped
>
> 1/2 teaspoon dried basil or 1 1/2 teaspoons fresh
>
> 1/2 teaspoon dried oregano
>
> 3 cups vegetable broth
>
> 1 10-ounce package frozen spinach, defrosted
>
> 1 28-ounce can crushed, peeled tomatoes
>
> 1 10-ounce can whole or chopped clams
>
> 8 ounces cooked pasta

Heat oil in a large soup pot over medium heat. Lower the heat and add onion and garlic. Cover and cook on low, stirring often, for 10 to 15 minutes or until the onion is translucent. Stir in the basil, oregano, broth, spinach, and tomatoes. Cook through on low for 5 to 10 minutes, or simmer up to 1 hour. Add the clams and cooked pasta. Heat for 3 minutes and serve.

Tomato, Spinach, and Bean Soup

6 servings—185 calories per serving

> 3 tablespoons olive oil
>
> 2 garlic cloves, peeled and chopped
>
> 1 medium onion, chopped

1 cup spinach, fresh or frozen (defrosted and drained)

1 19-ounce can cannellini beans, drained and rinsed

1 28-ounce can crushed tomatoes

4 cups chicken broth

1 teaspoon dried basil or 1 tablespoon fresh

1 teaspoon dried oregano or 1 tablespoon fresh

salt and pepper to taste

Heat oil in large pot over medium-low heat. Add garlic and onion and cook for 2 to 3 minutes or until garlic is golden and onion is translucent. Stir in seasonings. Add spinach and cook 3 minutes or until spinach is just wilted. Stir in tomatoes, chicken broth and beans. Heat through 3 to 5 minutes.

Note: Make extra spinach to use in spinach pocket sandwiches or another dinner this week.

Tomato, Spinach, and Bread Soup _____

10 servings—130 calories per serving

6 tablespoons olive oil

1/2 teaspoon crushed red pepper flakes (optional)

1 1/2 cups stale bread, cut into one-inch cubes

1 onion, diced

2 cloves garlic, peeled and finely chopped

1 cup spinach, fresh or frozen (defrosted and drained)

1 28-ounce can whole or crushed tomatoes

1 teaspoon dried basil

6 cups vegetable stock

salt and pepper to taste

Heat 4 tablespoons of oil in a large soup pot over medium-low heat. Stir in the red pepper flakes (if desired) and the bread.

Cook until the bread is golden, about 3 to 4 minutes, then remove to a plate and set aside. Add the remaining 2 tablespoons of oil to the pot, heat for 1 minute, and stir in the onion and garlic. Cook until onions and garlic are golden, about 10 minutes. Add the spinach and cook 3 minutes or until spinach is just wilted. Add the tomatoes, bread, and basil and simmer for about 15 minutes, stirring occasionally. Add the vegetable stock and bring to a boil. Reduce the heat to low and simmer for about 20 minutes. Add salt and pepper to taste and serve.

Dinners and Quick Sauces

Many of the following dinners are pasta-based. Remember to keep track of your pasta calories. If you are on a weight-loss meal plan, check it to see how much pasta to use. Most women should use 2 ounces of dry pasta (200 calories) which is about 1 cup of short, dry pasta. For men it's usually 3 ounces or about one 1 1/2 cups of short, dry pasta (300 calories). We encourage you to eat whole-wheat pasta; we think Delverde is the best tasting. If your store doesn't carry it, order it by calling 800–222–4409.

There are so many sauces and so little time, so make more sauce and freeze it for future use. But don't make more pasta than you need, or you may overeat or dip into it for a midnight snack.

If you need to eat a larger volume of food for dinner, increase the vegetables in a meal or sauce, but not the pasta or olive oil.

Baked Fish _____

2 servings—270 calories per serving

> 12 ounces white fish (see page 212)
> 2 tablespoons of olive oil
> fresh or dried herbs, such as bay leaves, basil, oregano,

and rosemary to taste black pepper, lemon juice, and
capers to taste (optional)

Preheat oven to 350 degrees. Place the fish in a baking pan and
brush or spoon the oil over the fish. Add the herbs, black pepper,
lemon juice, and capers if desired. Bake fish for 10 minutes per
inch of thickness.

Broiled Marinated Chicken Breast _____

2 servings—200 calories per serving

> 2 boneless, skinless chicken breasts (about 5 to 6
> ounces)
> 3/4 cup olive oil dressing (see page 204)

Place chicken breasts in a container and pour the dressing over,
completely coating the chicken with the dressing. Cover and
refrigerate, marinating the chicken at least 2 hours or overnight.
Preheat the broiler. Remove the marinated chicken from the
dressing and broil in roasting pan 4 to 5 minutes per side or until
chicken is cooked through. Serve with rice or potatoes and
greens, like spinach and broccoli.

*Note: An easy way to marinate is to put the chicken and the dressing in
a sealed plastic bag.*

Chicken Breasts Stuffed
with Spinach and Parmesan _____

2 servings—355 calories per serving

> 2 4-ounce chicken breasts
> 2 tablespoons olive oil
> 1 cup spinach or kale (frozen, cooked, or fresh)
> 4 basil leaves, chopped

4 tablespoons grated Parmesan or Romano cheese

pepper

Preheat oven to 400 degrees. Slice the chicken breast lengthwise halfway through the center, making a pocket. Heat the oil in a skillet over medium-low heat. Stir in the spinach or kale and basil. Cook about 3 minutes or until wilted. Remove from heat. Add cheese and stir to combine. Stuff mixture into chicken pockets. Secure chicken halves with oiled toothpicks. Lightly brush the top of the chicken with oil and sprinkle liberally with pepper. Bake for about 20 minutes or until chicken juices run clear. Remove toothpicks and serve.

Note: Use the extra spinach you made from the Tomato, Spinach, and Bean Soup for the chicken breasts in this recipe.

Chicken, Artichokes, Roasted Peppers, and Olives

2 servings—360 calories per serving

pepper to taste

4 to 6 tablespoons white flour

3 tablespoons olive oil

1 garlic clove, peeled and chopped

4 ounces chicken breast, cubed

2 roasted red peppers, from a jar, cut into strips

20 medium black olives

1 6-ounce jar marinated artichokes

Add black pepper to flour and roll the chicken cubes in the mixture to coat. Heat the oil in a large skillet over medium-low heat. Add the garlic and cook about 2 minutes. Add chicken and cook for about 4 minutes, turning until lightly browned on all sides. Add the peppers and olives and heat through, about 2 to 3 minutes. Add artichokes with liquid and cook until heated through, 3 more minutes. Serve over short pasta.

Note: This can be made without chicken by increasing the vegetables.

Frittata with Broccoli and Parmesan _____

Makes 1 single-serving frittata—475 calories per serving

>   2 teaspoons olive oil
>   2 tablespoons chopped onion
>   1 3/4 cups small pasta, cooked
>   1/3 cup chopped broccoli, fresh or frozen (defrosted)
>   2 tablespoons grated Parmesan or Romano cheese
>   1 tablespoon each fresh basil and oregano or 1 teaspoon dried
>   2 eggs

Preheat broiler. Coat 9-inch skillet with oil and heat on medium until oil is hot but not smoking, about 2 to 3 minutes. Add the onion and cook until golden. Add the pasta, broccoli, cheese, and herbs. Mix thoroughly. Pour eggs into skillet and spread around so the mixture covers the pan. Lower the heat to low and cook until set, about 5 minutes (the top should be semifirm). Remove from stovetop and place under the broiler. Broil until top is set and slightly browned, about 2 to 3 minutes. The top may brown quickly, so check after 1 minute.

Note: Make extra broccoli for use later in the week.

Frittata with Tomatoes and Potatoes _____

makes 1 single-serving frittata—440 calories per serving

4 teaspoons olive oil

2 fresh tomatoes or 1/4 cup canned, whole

2 tablespoons fresh basil, chopped

2 eggs, beaten

1/4 cup skim milk

3/4 cup potatoes, boiled and cubed

salt and pepper to taste

Preheat broiler. Heat the oil in a medium skillet over medium heat. Add the tomatoes and basil and cook about 2 to 3 minutes. Whisk eggs and milk in small bowl and add the potatoes, using a potato masher or fork to combine the egg and potatoes thoroughly. Add salt and pepper, if desired. Add the egg/potato mixture to the skillet and using a spatula, spread lightly and evenly. Cook on top of the stove until the mixture is semifirm, about 5 minutes. Put the pan under the broiler for about 3 minutes or until the top starts to brown. Use a spatula to loosen the mixture from the pan. Slide onto a plate and serve.

Garlic, Pine Nuts, and Red Peppers with Tomatoes and Olive Oil _____

2 servings—215 calories per serving

2 tablespoons olive oil

2 tablespoons pine nuts

2 medium garlic cloves, peeled and minced

1/2 cup roasted red peppers

2/3 cup canned tomatoes

pepper to taste

4 tablespoons fresh parsley

Heat olive oil in skillet on medium heat. Add pine nuts and garlic. Stir over medium heat until nuts and garlic are light brown, about 2 minutes. Add the roasted red peppers and heat another 2 minutes, stirring occasionally. Add the tomatoes and pepper. Continue to stir over medium heat until tomatoes are heated, about 3 minutes. Remove from heat and add parsley. Serve over short pasta.

Note: Jarred red peppers can be used for this recipe, but if you are roasting your own peppers make extra for sandwiches.

Mediterranean Beans and Red Sauce _____

2 servings—250 calories per serving

> 4 teaspoons olive oil
> 2 garlic cloves, peeled and minced
> 1 cup canned cannellini (white) beans, drained and
>   rinsed thoroughly
> 1/2 teaspoon basil
> 1/2 teaspoon oregano
> 1 cup canned crushed tomatoes or plain tomato sauce
> pepper to taste

Heat oil in medium saucepan over medium-high heat. Add the garlic and cook until golden, about 2 to 3 minutes. Stir in the spices. Add beans and heat through. Add tomatoes or sauce and stir to combine. Simmer for 3 more minutes. Serve over short pasta. Pepper to taste.

Mediterranean Clam Sauce _____

2 servings—180 calories per serving

> 4 teaspoons olive oil
> 2 garlic cloves, peeled and minced

red pepper flakes to taste

1 cup minced or chopped canned clams, drained (save
juice)

1 cup tomato sauce

pepper to taste

Optional:

1 cup spinach leaves

1/2 cup black olives, pitted and sliced

Heat oil in a medium saucepan over medium heat. Add garlic and red pepper flakes and reduce heat to medium low. Cook garlic until golden, 2 to 3 minutes. Add reserved clam juice, tomato sauce, and pepper. Stir and heat through, about 10 minutes. Add clams and cook about 3 more minutes. Serve over linguine or other long pasta.

Optional: Add spinach along with garlic and red pepper flakes and heat until wilted, 3 to 4 minutes; add olives at any point.

Mediterranean Grilled Salmon or Swordfish _____

2 servings—390 calories per serving

fresh or dried herbs like rosemary or oregano to taste

squeeze of fresh lemon

2 tablespoons olive oil

2 6-ounce swordfish or salmon steaks

Preheat broiler. Mix the herbs, lemon juice, and oil in a small bowl. Place the fish in a baking pan, brush the fish with the oil mixture, and broil for 5 minutes on both sides (10 minutes total per inch of thickness). Serve with rice or potatoes, and dark green, leafy vegetables like spinach or broccoli rabe.

Puttanesca Sauce _____

2 servings—230 calories per serving

> 4 teaspoons olive oil
>
> 2 garlic cloves, peeled and minced
>
> 1/4 teaspoon red pepper flakes
>
> 1 medium onion, chopped
>
> 4 ounces canned anchovy filets
>
> 20 black olives, pitted and sliced
>
> 4 tablespoons capers
>
> 1 tablespoon each fresh basil, oregano, and parsley or
>
>   2 teaspoons each dried
>
> 1 1/2 cups crushed, canned tomatoes
>
> pepper to taste

Heat oil in medium saucepan over medium-low heat. Reduce heat to low, add garlic, and stir for about 2 minutes. Garlic should be golden. Add red pepper flakes and stir for about 1 minute. Add onion and cook until translucent, 3 to 5 minutes. Add anchovies and break up with a fork. Add the olives, capers, herbs, and tomatoes. Stir. Cook 10 minutes, or continue cooking on low for up to 1 hour to blend flavors. Pepper to taste. Serve over pasta. This recipe can be made one day ahead and refrigerated.

Spicy Tomato Sauce _____

2 servings—255 calories per serving

> 4 teaspoons olive oil
>
> 2 garlic cloves, peeled and minced
>
> 1 teaspoon dried red pepper flakes

4 ounces canned anchovy filets, drained and chopped

2 cups crushed, canned tomatoes

20 black olives, chopped

2 tablespoons grated Parmesan or Romano cheese

Heat oil in medium saucepan over medium heat. Add garlic and red pepper flakes. Reduce heat to medium low and cook until garlic is golden, about 3 to 4 minutes. Add the anchovies and stir into the oil. Cook over medium-low heat about 3 to 4 minutes or until anchovies resemble a paste. Reduce heat to low. Add the tomatoes and olives. Heat through, about 3 to 4 minutes, or leave to simmer about 20 minutes (the extra time will allow the flavors to blend). Serve over pasta. Add cheese just before serving. Can be made ahead and refrigerated for one week, or it can be frozen up to two months.

Spicy Shrimp and Red Sauce

2 servings—290 calories per serving

2 tablespoons olive oil

2 garlic cloves, peeled and minced

1/2 teaspoon red pepper flakes

8 ounces fresh or frozen uncooked shrimp, peeled and deveined

1 cup crushed, canned tomatoes

Heat oil in skillet over medium-low heat. Add garlic and red pepper flakes and heat 2 to 3 minutes. Add shrimp and cook until shrimp is pink, about 3 to 4 minutes. Add tomato sauce or tomatoes and heat through, 3 minutes. Serve over pasta.

Spinach, Olives, and Red Pepper Sauce _____

2 servings—215 calories per serving

- 3 tablespoons olive oil
- 2 garlic cloves, peeled and minced
- 8 ounces frozen chopped spinach, defrosted and drained
- 20 olives, sliced
- 2 roasted red peppers, from jar

Heat oil in skillet over medium-low heat. Add garlic and cook for 2 to 3 minutes. Add spinach and stir to coat with oil. Cook 3 to 4 minutes. Add olives and roasted red peppers and heat through, about 3 to 4 minutes. Serve over short pasta.

Tuna, White Beans, and Olives in Tomato Sauce _____

2 servings—325 calories per serving

- 2 tablespoons olive oil
- 2 garlic cloves, peeled and minced
- 2/3 cup white (cannellini) beans, drained and rinsed
- 1 6-ounce can tuna packed in water, drained
- 20 black olives
- 1 cup crushed tomatoes
- 1 tablespoon fresh parsley, chopped

Heat oil in large skillet over medium heat. Add garlic and reduce heat to medium low, cooking until garlic is golden, about 3 to 4 minutes. Add beans and heat 2 to 3 minutes. Add tuna and heat 2 to 3 minutes. Stir in olives, tomatoes, and herbs. Heat through, 2 to 3 minutes. Serve over short pasta.

17 Losing Weight on the Mediterranean Diet

We have designed a weight-loss program using the healthy foods in the Mediterranean diet. Rich in high-fiber vegetables prepared in olive oil, the diet is filling yet low in calories. In order to roadtest the recipes and the meal plans, we offered the program to 120 people who came to Dr. Mary Flynn's Mediterranean diet weight-loss lectures at Brown University.

We then invited the attendees to be part of a focus group to determine (1) if they lost weight, (2) if the diet was easy to follow, and (3) if the diet satisfied their hunger.

We studied the focus group participants for eight weeks, communicating with them through e-mail several times a week and encouraging them to contact us with any questions, comments, and suggestions. All of the participants reported steady weight loss, and many indicated they did so without being hungry. After eight weeks, the weight loss ranged from six to thirteen pounds, with an average of just over eight pounds. Following are some of their comments:

Restaurant Dining and Weight Loss

The problem with eating out at restaurants is that generally the portions served are far too generous for the average person—and many of us tend to overorder. The key to weight loss is portion control. Here are a few tips for keeping your weight under control even when eating out.

- When eating at home, notice what a normal portion looks like so you can compare it to a restaurant portion. For instance, train your eye to recognize what two or three ounces of pasta looks like on your plate, and then stick to the limits you establish for yourself.

- Instead of ordering an entree, order two or three appetizers and share them. Or order one appetizer and share the entree. It's a great way to explore a variety of tastes and to keep portions under control.

- Use restaurants to explore the wonderful world of soups—especially soups that are vegetable-based as opposed to cream-based.

- Look for salads made with dark greens like spinach and arugula. Iceberg lettuce is a less desirable salad choice, especially if you want to maximize phytochemicals and nutrients in your diet.

- Try to get your weekly quota of fish (aim for two fish dishes a week) by eating it when you dine out. This way, you won't have to worry about where to purchase fresh fish, and you'll be getting your intake of healthy omega-3 fatty acids.

"I had never used olive oil before and I'm sorry that I spent all those years not enjoying its delicious taste. I am never hungry between meals...."

"I am surprised to discover that potatoes with olive oil taste just as good to me as with butter or margarine.... "

"This is the best (and easiest) diet I have ever tried."

"Thank you for... introducing me to this comfortable and sensible way to lose weight."

Meal Plans for a Mediterranean Diet

The meal plans that follow are guides to help you start incorporating Mediterranean foods into your diet and lose weight. The 1,500-calorie meal plan is for women and the 2,000-calorie meal plan is for men. The meals are drawn from the list of recipes starting on page 198. Try one of the following meal plans for a few days and see how you feel. If you are experiencing extreme hunger, add 200 to 300 calories, preferably vegetables and fruits. If you have not lost at least one pound after a week, reduce your calorie level. If you want more personal guidance in using the Mediterranean diet for weight loss or would like to give us feedback, visit our website at *www.med-diet.com*.

Meal Plan for a 1,500 Calorie Diet

This calorie level is for most women or smaller, sedentary men.

DAY 1: 1,500 CALORIES

Breakfast:

Breakfast of choice between 250 and 300 calories (page 202)

Lunch:

Spinach Pocket (see page 209)

1 medium fruit

Dinner:

Baked Fish (see page 216)

Mediterranean Mashed Potatoes (see page 210)

1 cup broccoli

Salad: 1 cup mixed greens and 1 tablespoon Basic Olive Oil
Dressing (see page 204)

1 fruit

DAY 2: 1,500 CALORIES

Breakfast:

Breakfast of choice between 250 and 300 calories (see page
202)

Lunch:

Cheese and Roasted Red Pepper Sandwich (see page 204)

1 fruit

Dinner:

Chicken, Artichokes, Roasted Peppers, and Olives (see page
218)

1 cup pasta (dry weight)

1 fruit

DAY 3: 1,500 CALORIES

Breakfast:

Breakfast of choice between 250 and 300 calories (see page
202)

Lunch:

Italian Potato Salad (see page 205)

1 slice bread

1 fruit

Dinner:

Tuna, White Beans, and Olives in Tomato Sauce (see page 225)

1 1/2 cups pasta (dry weight)

Salad with 1 tablespoon Basic Olive Oil Dressing (see page 204)

DAY 4: 1,500 CALORIES

Breakfast:

Breakfast of choice between 250 and 300 calories (see page 202)

Lunch:

Peppers, Mushrooms, and Onion Pocket (see page 208)

1 slice bread

1 fruit

Dinner:

Spinach, Olives, and Red Peppers (see page 225)

1 1/2 cups pasta (dry weight)

2 slices bread

1 fruit

Salad with 1 tablespoon Basic Olive Oil Dressing (see page 204)

DAY 5: 1,500 CALORIES

Breakfast:

Breakfast of choice between 250 and 300 calories (page 202)

Lunch:

Mediterranean Bean Salad (see page 206)

1 slice bread

1 fruit

Dinner:

Spicy Shrimp and Red Sauce (see page 224)

1 cup cooked rice (made with 1 teaspoon olive oil)

1 fruit

Salad with 1 tablespoon Basic Olive Oil Dressing (see page 204)

DAY 6: 1,500 CALORIES

Breakfast:

Breakfast of choice between 250 and 300 calories (see page 202)

Lunch:

Italian Tuna Salad (see page 205)

greens and vegetables

1 slice bread

1 fruit

Dinner:

Chicken Breasts Stuffed with Spinach and Parmesan (see page 217)

large baked potato with 2 teaspoons olive oil

1 fruit

DAY 7: 1,500 CALORIES

Breakfast:

Breakfast of choice between 250 and 300 calories (page 202)

Lunch:

Italian Pasta Salad (see page 205)

1 slice bread

1 medium fruit

Dinner:

Frittata with Tomatoes and Potatoes (see page 219)

Mixed greens and vegetable salad with 1 tablespoon Basic
    Olive Oil Dressing (see page 204)

1 fruit

Meal Plan for a 2,000 Calorie Diet

This calorie level is for most men who want to lose weight. Adjust
this diet according to your individual needs.

DAY 1: 2,000 CALORIES

Breakfast:

Breakfast of choice between 300 and 400 calories (see page
    202)

Lunch:

Spinach Pocket (see page 209)

1 fruit

Salad with 2 tablespoons Basic Olive Oil Dressing (see page
    204)

Dinner:

Baked Fish (see page 216)

Mediterranean Mashed Potatoes (see page 210)

1 cup broccoli

Salad of 1 cup lettuce and 2 tablespoons Basic Olive Oil
    Dressing (see page 204)

1 fruit

DAY 2: 2,000 CALORIES

Breakfast:

Breakfast of choice between 300 and 400 calories (page 202)

Lunch:

Cheese and Roasted Red Pepper Sandwich (see page 204)

1 fruit

Dinner:

Chicken, Artichokes, Roasted Peppers, and Olives (see page 218)

1 1/2 cups pasta (dry weight)

2 slices bread

1 fruit

Salad with 2 tablespoons Basic Olive Oil Dressing (see page 204)

DAY 3: 2,000 CALORIES

Breakfast:

Breakfast of choice between 300 and 400 calories (see page 202)

Lunch:

Italian Potato Salad (see page 205)

greens

2 slices bread

1 medium fruit

Dinner:

Tuna, White Beans, and Olives in Tomato Sauce (see page 225)

1 1/2 cups pasta (dry weight)

2 slices bread

1 fruit

Salad with 2 tablespoons Basic Olive Oil Dressing (see page 204)

DAY 4: 2,000 CALORIES

Breakfast:

Breakfast of choice between 300 and 400 calories (see page 202)

Lunch:

Peppers, Mushrooms, and Onion Pocket (see page 208)

1 fruit

Salad with 2 tablespoons Basic Olive Oil Dressing (see page 204)

Dinner:

Spinach, Olives, and Red Peppers (see page 225)

2 cups pasta (dry weight)

2 slices bread with 2 teaspoons spread

1 fruit

Salad with 2 tablespoons Basic Olive Oil Dressing (page 204)

DAY 5: 2,000 CALORIES

Breakfast:

Breakfast of choice between 300 and 400 calories (see page 202)

Lunch:

Mediterranean Bean Salad (see page 206)

2 slices bread

1 fruit

Dinner:

Spicy Shrimp and Red Sauce (see page 224)

1 cup rice (cooked with 2 teaspoons olive oil)

2 slices bread

1 fruit

Salad with 2 tablespoons Basic Olive Oil Dressing (see page 204)

DAY 6: 2,000 CALORIES

Breakfast:

Breakfast of choice between 300 and 400 calories (see page 202)

Lunch:

Italian Tuna Salad (see page 205)

2 slices bread

1 fruit

Dinner:

Chicken Breast Stuffed with Spinach (see page 217)

1 large baked potato with 1 tablespoon olive oil

1 slice bread

1 fruit

Salad with 2 tablespoons Basic Olive Oil Dressing (page 204)

DAY 7: 2,000 CALORIES

Breakfast:

Breakfast of choice between 300 and 400 calories (see page 202)

Lunch:

Italian Pasta Salad (see page 205)

2 slices bread

1 fruit

Dinner:

Frittata with Tomatoes and Potatoes (see page 219)

2 slices bread

Salad with 2 tablespoons Basic Olive Oil Dressing (see page 204)

1 fruit

18 Walk Like an Italian

It's hard to lose weight and keep it off without some exercise. But exercise does not need to be painful; it can be something you look forward to. Walking is probably the single best exercise you can do. And, just as with food, Mediterraneans have elevated walking to an art form. Indeed the simple act of walking and talking is both a ceremony and a social institution that is at the core of Italian life. It is a source of exercise, fellowship, relaxation, communication, psychotherapy, street theater, and pure amusement. It is one of the many features of the Mediterranean life that makes it so healthy. If we walked like the Italians we would be much healthier.

The *passeggiata*, or the walk, is as much a part of Italian life as olive oil, tomato sauce, and red wine. The passeggiata starts every afternoon at around 4 o'clock, and by 5 o'clock it is in full swing as Italians take to the streets. From the small towns to the big cities, the scene is the same as young lovers, old friends, and new acquaintances walk together, often arm in arm, down the main streets and piazzas. As they stroll and window shop, political affairs of the day are discussed, business deals are made, courtships are begun, gossip is embellished, infatuations are stoked, and heated arguments are resolved or started. Those who walk create a wonderful spectacle for those who watch.

Unfortunately the rhythm of our workday and our daily commute don't lend themselves to this communal celebration, and it would be hard to re-create the same sight in a suburban setting. However, that doesn't mean we can't learn something from the passeggiata and in some way incorporate its lesson in our own lives. The most basic message is that we need to exercise, and the simplest, most valuable, most enjoyable exercise is walking. It is a fundamental human activity that we enjoyed long before the car, elevator, TV, and Internet.

There are two reasons why obesity and the metabolic syndrome are epidemic in America: We eat too much and exercise too little. Many Americans go months without any significant physical activity. We get up, drive to work, park as close to the front door as possible, take the elevator upstairs, and sit at our desks until we walk down the hall to a meeting, where we sit until it's time to take the elevator down to the cafeteria for lunch. At the end of a day of sitting, we drive home, hit the garage door opener, and head inside. The pizza guy delivers dinner, and then we grab the remote and click on the TV until it's time to go to bed. In the morning we get dressed, and as we look in the mirror we wonder why we have put on twenty pounds. Then we get in our car and start our sedentary day all over again.

From 1960 to the late 1970s, obesity in America increased

Kill Your TV Before It Kills You

The first step toward incorporating exercise into your life is to eliminate those influences that stop you from exercising in the first place. Most of us say we don't exercise because we don't have time. But the average American spends seven hours a day watching TV. Even if you are not one of these TV addicts, chances are you spend an hour or two in front of the TV three or four days a week. In the time it takes to watch one sitcom, you could get in your quota of brisk walking for the day.

If you can't bring yourself to kill your TV, you have to at least get control of it. As with food you have to get a sense of portion size—if you don't, TV will kill you. Budget your time in front of the TV and the computer and get moving. If you don't, someday you may be watching TV in a hospital coronary care unit with the Grim Reaper lurking at your door.

about 4.5 percent, but from the late seventies to 1991 it increased 31 percent. What produced this explosion in obesity? As you might expect, there are several causes: Low-fat diets have become the law of the dietary land, and as people consume low-fat foods with abandon, sugar consumption has gone through the roof, as have total calories. Fast-food chains have multiplied, and our lives have become more sedentary. Cable started coming into homes in the 1980s and is now almost ubiquitous. Nielsen ratings report that hours of TV watching have gone up at least 15 percent since the mid-1970s. Almost no one had a computer in the 1970s, but now it seems as though almost everyone has one. Rather than walking and talking with a friend, we interact with each other through the Internet. Our children spend hours watching TV, then spend several more hours playing video games.

And don't be deluded by the booming sneaker business. Despite steep sales in running shoes, the number of serious exercisers has remained pretty much constant for the past decade. Even if you don't want to lose weight, you have to get moving if you want to be healthy.

Exerting the will to exert yourself is not easy. On top of our culture of convenience, the pressures of work and family seem to conspire against us. But there is hope. There are ways to get moving without quitting your job, abandoning your loved ones, and moving into the gym. To get moving you have to weave walking and movement into your life so that it becomes as habitual as the passeggiata in Italy. It may not be part of American culture, but it can become the culture of your family and a few of your friends. By embedding your diet and your walking into your personal culture and the culture of your friends and family, your maximize your chances for long-term success.

The Mediterranean diet is an extraordinarily healthy diet, and as a culturally based, harmonious, time-tested cuisine, we think it is a way of purchasing, preparing, and consuming food that you will find easier to live with over the long haul. But to maximize its benefit and to enhance your ability to stick with this new way of choosing and consuming food, exercise is very important. Exercise is helpful not only because it burns calories but also because, as research shows, it helps people stick with other lifestyle changes, including even smoking programs. Those who exercise, usually by brisk walking, have more success sticking to diets. It's not clear whether this success is the result of the commitment to healthier living in general, exercise's beneficial effect on mood, or other factors. But we know that people who decide to walk or exercise make better choices when confronted with the temptation to overeat.

And exercise has yet another benefit in aiding weight loss: It suppresses hunger.

The next time you're feeling hungry and looking for a snack, go for a brisk walk or do something else that gets your pulse up and makes you break a sweat. You will find that your hunger will abate and will stay suppressed for a while after you exercise. When you exercise, blood flow to the intestines is diminished as blood flow to the muscles is increased. As your body makes that shift, it moves from an energy-storage mode to an energy-expenditure mode. Although hunger plays an integral role in the energy-storage mode, it is of little use in the expenditure or activity mode and is temporarily suppressed. But does hunger then return with a vengeance and cause us to overconsume, nullifying the benefits of exercise? Research suggests that for most overweight people, this is not the case. Usually, we come out ahead when we exercise.

As we have been using the word "exercise," you may have had painful or embarrassing flashbacks to a gym class; intimidating images of intricate exercise machinery in expensive gyms; or visions of mindless, endless, automated stair climbing. While there is nothing wrong with gym workouts if that's your pleasure, they are certainly not for everybody. And even a forty-five-minute workout turns into an hour and a half when you factor in traveling, parking, changing, showering, and dressing again. Even people who have the time and the inclination to go to the gym two or three times a week would benefit from weaving increased walking into their way of life.

Below are some recommendations to get you moving with a minimum of pain and inconvenience. It's important to choose activities you will enjoy and to start slowly. It is much better to be consistent with fifteen minutes of activity seven days a week and slowly build up the time and level of exertion than to erratically engage in forty minutes of movement once or twice a week. As with wine, a little bit of exercise every day is far more beneficial than a large amount every Saturday. Of course, if you have heart disease or other serious medical conditions, you should check with your doctor before engaging in an exercise program.

The Morning Passeggiata

Once the day gets going we seem to lose control of it as the unexpected crops up. The last-minute conference call wipes out your plans to take a fifteen-minute walk at lunchtime, and the deadline you have to meet tomorrow means you have to work late tonight. Tomorrow you have a business dinner and the night after that your child's soccer game. The answer is to get a walk in before the day gets going. The morning is the time of day when you have the most control. All of us can get up a half-hour earlier, slip on our sneakers, walk fifteen minutes in one direction and fifteen minutes back. When you come back, take the shower you were going to take anyway and get ready for work.

You say you're not a morning person. You don't have to shock your body with joint-pounding jogging first thing in the morning. Just walk slowly at first and pick up speed as you warm up. By the time you get back, you will feel great and have a stress relieving natural high that will carry through the day. If you do this seven days a week, you will lose weight, be happier, and live longer.

Don't worry if you blow it sometimes. A ten-minute walk is great. Remember you can make up for it later in the day because your thirty or forty-five minutes a day doesn't have to be all at the same time. Research has shown that thirty minutes of intermittent exercise is just as effective as thirty minutes of continuous exercise as long as the segments are about eight to ten minutes in length. And

Walk Through the Mediterranean Diet Pyramid

Unlike the USDA food pyramid, the Mediterranean diet pyramid, developed by Oldways Preservation and Trust, not only is a valuable guide to healthy eating but also includes exercise. It recognizes that exercise, like red wine and olive oil, is an intrinsic part of the Mediterranean way of life. The message is don't just eat your way through the pyramid, walk it, too (see Mediterranean diet pyramid on page 145).

if you miss a day, don't throw in the towel. Five or six days of walking a week is infinitely better than none. If you prefer, you can walk a half-hour a day, five days a week, then do an hour-and-a-half hike on Saturday, and an hour on Sunday. How you schedule it is up to you. The most important thing is that you exercise every day—make it part of your daily routine, just like brushing your teeth.

If you walk thirty minutes a day you will improve your health and probably lose weight—for the average person, forty-five minutes of brisk walking daily (a rate of about four miles an hour) virtually guarantees significant weight loss. Although you still can't pig out at mealtimes, the extra three hundred calories you'll burn each day will allow you to be less obsessive about counting calories.

The Rest of the Day

Because the effect of exercise is cumulative, you should develop strategies to get ten- to fifteen-minute blocks of exercise throughout the day. Instead of parking as close to the front door as possible, find a safe place to park a few blocks away so you have a ten-minute walk to work. At the end of the day, or if you have an outside meeting, it's another ten minutes back to the car. That's another twenty more minutes of activity for the day. It doesn't sound like a lot, but that's one hundred minutes over the course of a five-day workweek. It adds up.

If you get an hour for lunch, devote fifteen minutes of it to walking. It's great if you can walk with a coworker. Maybe you can find a deli nearby that makes great grilled vegetables. Walk there instead of eating the same old cafeteria food.

Never take the elevator. Climb the stairs. When I lived in Italy twenty years ago, our apartment building had a rickety elevator that seemed to be perpetually broken. All of us had to go up and down the stairs two, four, or sometimes six times a day. I was always amazed at the stamina of the older ladies who lived upstairs. After watching them go up and down, I have no doubt that a lifetime of stair climbing adds years to your life. People pay lots of money to use a Stairmaster. Save your money; just take the stairs.

Even if you walked in the morning, try to squeeze in some exercise to perk you up at the end of the day. If you have no time to do anything fancy, go for another walk. This is often the best time to share a walk with someone else, such as your spouse. Walking and talking at the end of the day ensures quality time without distraction. Not only is it good for your health and spirit, it feeds your relationship as well. And research shows that healthy relationships go hand in hand with a healthy, long life.

The moral is walk, walk, and walk some more. Life is a journey, and much of it should be traveled on foot.

Other Activities You Can Do

A daily walk may require a little effort and may at first seem more like an obligation than recreation, but stick to it and you will soon look forward to it. Still, there are other activities you can do to get exercise into your life with enjoyment. Here are a few examples:

Ride a bike. Biking is great exercise because there is limited stress on the joints and you get to explore your surroundings. Don't worry if you haven't biked in years. It's true that once you learn how to ride a bike you never forget how. If you need to shop for a bike, don't be intimidated by what you see in bike stores these days. You don't need something with a titanium frame and twenty-seven gears. You can get a perfectly good bike for less than $200— less if you buy it used. Make sure that the bike you choose has good brakes—and wear a helmet. Then join a bike club. Not only do bike clubs chart out weekly trips on safe roads, they are also a great way to meet new friends. Bike clubs often do tours on Sunday mornings. Clubs are always looking for new members, and novices are welcome.

Take dancing lessons. I can't think of a better activity than dancing. It's fun, social, low impact, and a great workout. Don't worry if you don't know how to dance; now is the time to learn. Salsa and swing are in. Both are fast dances that really work up a sweat, and in one or two lessons you can get the basics down. If you have a partner, great. If you don't, that's not a problem; there are always unpaired beginners to practice with at dance studios. Once again, its a great way to get out of the house and meet new people.

Gardening. You might not think of gardening as vigorous activity, but the constant hand motion, bending, stooping, and digging keep you moving and are very good for you. The time passes quickly, and you get a tangible payoff—beautiful flowers, or perhaps vegetables you can eat. Gardening is also a great way to relieve stress and get back to nature. There is nothing as satisfying as growing your own tomatoes and basil and using them to make a delicious salad. Growing your own food helps you develop a reverence for it and the environment.

Coach a team. Coach any team—little league football, soccer, baseball, T-ball, ice hockey, field hockey, or lacrosse—it doesn't matter. Don't know that much about sports? Just coach a young age group (just getting them to line up straight may be the most sophisticated part of the job). This is a chance for you to run around with the kids, play with them, and encourage them. You just can't have any more fun than this.

Go hiking. Hiking is walking taken to the next level. It's vigorous, visually stimulating, and spiritually satisfying. Hours can go by without your even realizing it. Hiking is great to do with a soul mate or with a group of people. Once again there are probably hiking clubs in your area that can give you information about the best trails and introduce you to people with similar interests.

Get a dog, and walk it. Owning a dog is associated with better health. Dogs are great companions and do wonders for those who are otherwise isolated or alone. Petting a dog is said to lower blood pressure. Of course a dog is also a good excuse to get some exercise. If you walk briskly and train your dog not to stop every two feet, a dog can be a great workout companion that can nag you on those mornings you're feeling a little lazy. They are creatures of habit, and they will help you stick to your routine.

Mentor a child. There are thousands of kids looking for a role model and an adult to spend time with them. The need is especially acute in the inner cities. I can't think of a better way to change a child's life and feed your own soul than by mentoring. But don't take your child to McDonalds; play catch, kick a ball around, go for a hike, go ice skating, or go for a walk on the beach. It will be good for you as well as the child.

These are just a few ideas. There are hundreds of things you can do from bowling to bocce to snowboarding to inline skating. But the key is to do something physical every day. So even if you are an avid weekend hiker, biker, dancer, or gardener, keep moving during the week.

It may be hard to find a friend to walk with every morning, but try to involve friends in some of your other activities. It is the companionship and the conversation that makes the Mediterranean passeggiata so rich, healthy, and joyful. Not only does companionship make any activity more fun, making it more likely that you will stick with it, but it is very important to emotional and physical health. There is a good deal of research to show that those who are socially isolated or depressed have a significantly higher rate of death from heart disease. This is one of the great lessons of the Mediterranean lifestyle. The emphasis on family, friends, and community is as important as the emphasis on food and exercise.

To be truly healthy you cannot merely eat well and exercise— you must feed your soul. You must engage yourself in the lives of others and in the life of your community. You may have to work at it. But it's worth it. Because really, that's what life is all about, and that's the most valuable thing we can learn from the Mediterranean way of life.

19 Mediterranean Recipes from American Restaurants

In the following pages we provide recipes from a variety of restaurants across the country, including my family's restaurant, Christopher Martins, in New Haven, Connecticut. All the chefs have made their recipe contributions with the Mediterranean theme in mind. Although somewhat more complicated than Flynn's recipes, most of these can be tackled by the novice. These restaurant recipes tend to be higher in calories, so adjust portion sizes according to your personal needs.

Each recipe has been selected to provide you with a taste of the Mediterranean as well as healthy Mediterranean nutrients, especially olive oil. Many of these recipes can be made with minor additions to the list of basic ingredients that form the foundation of your new Mediterranean lifestyle—in America.

Brunch and Light Lunch

Panzanella _____

From Legal Sea Foods, Inc., Burlington, MA; Chestnut Hill, MA; Boston, MA; Prudential, MA; Cambridge, MA; Natick, MA; Peabody, MA; Nyack, NY; Warwick, RI; Washington, DC; McLean, VA

Executive chef: Richard Vellante

4 servings—466 calories per serving

> 8 ounces stale or day-old hearth bread, remove crusts
>   and cube into 3/4-inch pieces
> 1/4 cup chicken stock or water
> 2 large ripe tomatoes, seeded and diced
> 1 large red onion, sliced thin
> 2 cucumbers, seeded and diced into 1/2-inch pieces
> 1 cup kalamata olives, pitted and coarsely chopped
> 3/4 cup loosely packed basil leaves, coarsely chopped
> 1/2 cup extra-virgin olive oil
> 1/4 cup red wine vinegar
> salt and pepper to taste

Moisten bread with chicken stock or water (remove the excess liquid and be careful not to overmoisten bread.) Combine the tomatoes, onion, cucumbers, olives, and bread in a bowl and fold in basil. Moisten mixture with olive oil and red wine vinegar (you may not need all of the oil or vinegar). Salt and pepper to taste. Thoroughly mix to blend ingredients. Set aside in a cool spot for 30 minutes to allow flavors to develop (do not refrigerate).

Spanish Potato and Vegetable Omelet
(Tortilla de Legumbres) _____

From Cafe Ba-Ba-Reeba!, Chicago, IL

8 servings—344 calories per serving

> 1 cup olive oil
> 2 medium potatoes, peeled and cut into small cubes
> 1 medium onion, chopped
> 1 medium red pepper, chopped
> 1/4 cup cooked lima beans
> 1/4 cup cooked peas
> 4 large eggs

Heat the olive oil in a medium-sized skillet. Add the potatoes, onion, and pepper and cook over medium heat until tender. Drain the vegetables, reserving about 8 tablespoons of oil in the skillet. Add beans and peas and sauté. Drain, but save the oil. Beat the eggs in a large bowl and add all the vegetables. Pour the olive oil back into the skillet and add the egg mixture. Use a spatula to pull back the outside edge of the omelet, allowing the egg mixture to flow underneath. When the omelet is brown underneath, turn and cook until brown on the other side. Place on plate and garnish with chopped parsley when cool. The omelet may be sliced or cut into squares and served with frill picks. This dish is served at room temperature in Spain.

Spanish Tortilla of Greens and Potatoes _____

From Tosca, Hingham, MA
Chef: Joe Simone

A cousin of the Italian frittata, this dish is a staple of Catalan, the north-

east part of Spain centering around Barcelona. This tortilla can be served piping hot or, as is the custom in Spain, at room temperature. This dish can be made with leftover vegetables, so let your imagination be your guide.

4 to 6 servings—385-255 (respectively) calories per serving

3 tablespoons extra-virgin olive oil

2 garlic cloves, minced

2 packed cups escarole, washed and chopped

1 packed cup spinach, washed and chopped

kosher salt to taste

1 cup Spanish onions, chopped

2 large Yukon Gold potatoes, boiled

6 eggs, beaten

1/2 cup grated Parmesan cheese (optional)

freshly ground black pepper and kosher salt to taste

Preheat oven to 350 degrees. Heat 1 1/2 tablespoons of oil in a large, heavy-bottomed skillet over medium-high heat. Add the garlic and greens and stir to combine. Season the greens with salt and continue cooking until the greens give off their liquid and begin to wilt, about 3 to 4 minutes. Remove from heat, drain greens well, and set aside. Heat the remaining olive oil in a medium-sized nonstick skillet. Add the onions and cook until translucent, about 7 minutes. Add the cooked greens and potatoes and stir to combine. Add the eggs and stir as if you were making scrambled eggs. When the eggs are beginning to set, stir in the cheese, if desired, and continue stirring until the eggs are partially set. Place the skillet in the preheated oven and cook for 15 to 20 minutes until the eggs are thoroughly set, but not too dry. Remove the skillet from the oven and serve immediately or allow to cool and serve with a small salad. Add freshly ground black pepper and kosher salt to taste.

Spicy Tuna, Caper, Anchovy, and Tomato Sandwiches

Flea Street Cafe, Palo Alto, CA
Chef: Jessie Cool

4 servings—270 calories per serving

> 1 large can water-packed tuna, drained
> 1/4 cup red onion, finely minced
> 1/2 cup celery or fennel bulb, finely chopped
> 1 1/2 tablespoons capers
> 2 tablespoons chopped anchovy filets
> 2 hard-boiled eggs, grated
> 2 tablespoons finely chopped parsley
> 2 tablespoons or more olive oil to moisten
> 1/2 teaspoon red pepper flakes
> 8 slices vine-ripened tomatoes
> 8 slices bread

Place tuna in a medium bowl and combine with the red onion, celery, capers, anchovies, grated eggs, and parsley. Add enough olive oil to moisten thoroughly. Add red pepper flakes. Place tomatoes on one piece of bread. Season with salt and pepper. Place a generous amount of tuna salad on top. Top with the other piece of bread. Makes four sandwiches with some tuna salad left over for lunch the next day!

Chicken Noodle Soup _____

Christopher Martins, New Haven, CT

Chef: Mary Melie

8 servings—146 calories per serving

> 1 tablespoon olive oil
>
> 1 tablespoon garlic, chopped
>
> 1 large onion, chopped
>
> 2 medium carrots, chopped
>
> 6 stalks celery, chopped
>
> 1/2 pound cooked chicken, cubed
>
> 1/4 cup dry white wine
>
> 1 1/2 quarts chicken stock
>
> salt and pepper to taste
>
> 6 tablespoons parsley, chopped
>
> 1 tablespoon chopped thyme
>
> 4 ounces dry noodles (or any cooked pasta)

Heat the oil in a large pot over medium heat. Add the garlic, vegetables, and chicken and reduce heat. Cook for about 5 minutes. When vegetables start to change color, add wine and stock. Bring to a boil and reduce heat to simmer. Simmer for 20 minutes. Season with salt, pepper, parsley, and thyme. Serve hot.

Potato and Leek Soup _____

Christopher Martins, New Haven, CT

Chef: Mary Melie

8 servings—136 calories per serving

> 2 pounds russet potatoes, peeled and cubed
>
> 1 leek (white part only), chopped

1 teaspoon garlic, chopped

2 quarts chicken stock

2 cups 1%-low-fat milk

salt and pepper to taste

1 teaspoon fresh chives, chopped

In a medium pot, barely cover potatoes, leek, and garlic with stock and simmer over low heat, about 1 hour. When vegetables are tender, add any remaining stock and milk and simmer for about 5 minutes. Add salt and pepper to taste. Carefully purée half of the soup in the blender, then mix together. Serve hot with garnish of chives.

Roasted Eggplant and Garlic Soup _____

Christopher Martins, New Haven, CT

Chef: Mary Melie

6 servings—93 calories per serving

1 medium eggplant (about 1 1/4 cups)

1 tablespoon olive oil

1 small onion, diced

4 garlic cloves, roasted (see page 285)

1/2 cup white wine

4 cups chicken stock

salt and pepper to taste

2 tablespoons fresh basil, chopped

3 plum tomatoes, diced

croutons

Preheat oven to 400 degrees. Place the eggplant in a small roasting pan. Roast for about 25 minutes or until soft to the touch. Remove the eggplant to a paper bag and let cool 10 minutes. Heat oil in

medium saucepan over medium heat and add the onion and garlic. Cook until the onion is translucent, 3 to 5 minutes. Add 1/4 cup
of the white wine. Peel the eggplant and dice the remaining pulp,
add to pot, and cook for 3 minutes. Add the stock and bring to a
boil. Reduce the heat to simmer. Season with salt and pepper. Stir
in the basil and tomatoes. Serve with croutons.

Soupa Faki

Taverna Cretekou, Alexandria, VA
Chef: George Maltabes

*During the Lenten season, this legume soup is popular fare. Serve with
fresh bread and boiled greens dressed with olive oil and lemon juice.*

6 servings—268 calories per serving

> 1 pound lentils, rinsed and picked over
> 1/4 cup olive oil
> 2 medium onions, chopped
> 3 stalks celery, chopped
> 2 small carrots, chopped
> 2 cloves garlic, minced
> 2 tablespoons tomato paste
> 2 bay leaves
> 1 tablespoon fresh oregano, minced, or 1 teaspoon
>   dried, crushed
> salt and freshly ground pepper, to taste
> 1/2 cup red wine or red wine vinegar to taste

Boil lentils for 10 minutes, then discard water. Warm oil in a large,
heavy-bottomed stockpot over medium heat. Add onions, celery,
carrots, garlic, tomato paste, bay leaves, and oregano. Sauté until
onions are translucent, about 5 minutes. Add lentils and water to

cover by about 3 inches. Bring to a boil, cover, reduce heat, and simmer until lentils are tender, about 30 minutes. Check periodically to make sure the lentils are completely covered with water, adding more if necessary. Remove bay leaves. Season with salt, pepper, and wine. Cover and let stand a few minutes to blend flavors, then serve.

Tuscan Bean Soup

The University Club, Providence, RI
Chef: Gary Camella

10 servings—266 calories per serving

- 1 pound cannellini beans, rinsed, picked over, and soaked overnight
- 8 tablespoons olive oil
- 2 cups fresh fennel, chopped into 1/4-inch pieces
- 2 large onions, chopped into 1/4-inch pieces
- 2 carrots, peeled and diced
- 1 tablespoon garlic, chopped
- 1 teaspoon sea salt
- 1 bay leaf
- 1 teaspoon crushed red pepper flakes
- 1 small head green cabbage, shredded
- 2 cups Roma tomatoes, peeled, seeded, and diced
- 1/4 cup tomato paste
- grated parmesan cheese

Place the beans in a large stockpot with 4 quarts of water. Bring to a boil, reduce heat, and simmer until the beans are cooked, but not mushy, about 1 to 1 1/2 hours. Heat 4 tablespoons of olive oil in a large pan over medium heat. Add the fennel, onion, carrots, garlic, and salt. Sauté until vegetables are soft and wilted, about 10 minutes. Add the bay leaf, red pepper flakes, and cabbage and sauté 5 minutes. Add the beans to the vegetables and add stock to a desired consistency. Reduce heat to low, stir in the tomato paste and cook 10 to 15 minutes, stirring often. The soup should be slightly thickened. Adjust the seasonings and serve piping hot, drizzled with remaining olive oil and sprinkled with parmesan cheese.

Pisto Manchégo Vegetable Stew "La Manchis" Style

Iberia Restaurant, Portola Valley, CA

Chef/owner: Jose Luis Relinque

4 servings—460 calories per serving

> 1/2 cup olive oil
> 2 large potatoes, diced and soaked in cold water
> salt to taste
> 2 large onions, coarsely chopped
> 3 large bell peppers (green, red, or both)
> 3 medium tomatoes, coarsely chopped
> 2 medium zucchini, diced
> 4 eggs
> pinch saffron threads

Drain potatoes and pat dry. Preheat oven to 375 degrees. Heat olive oil in large skillet over medium heat. Sprinkle potatoes with salt and brown on all sides. Add onions and peppers and cook until lightly browned, about 3 to 5 minutes. Add tomatoes and saffron. Cook to reduce liquid to desired consistency. Add zucchini and cook until tender, about 3 to 5 minutes. Season to taste. To serve, portion out into four ramekins. Make an indentation in the middle and break an egg in each. Bake until egg is set to taste.

Salads and Dressings

Melitzanosalata (Eggplant Salad) _____

Taverna Opa, Hollywood, FL
Chef: Giorgio Bakatsias

4 servings—83 calories per serving

> 1 large eggplant
> 1 small red pepper, roasted (see recipe on page 286)
> 2 garlic cloves, peeled and minced
> 1 small onion, roasted and chopped
> 1/4 teaspoon dried oregano
> 1/4 teaspoon ground cumin (optional)
> 1–2 teaspoons lemon juice
> 2 tablespoons extra-virgin olive oil
> salt and freshly ground pepper to taste
> chopped parsley
> crusty bread, flatbread, or pita chips

Preheat oven to 350 degrees. Place the eggplant on a baking sheet, pierce it with a fork, and bake 20 to 30 minutes until the pulp is soft. Or, you may grill the eggplant along with the peppers. Put the eggplant in a paper bag for a few minutes to loosen the skin. Skin, stem, and dice finely. In a food processor or blender, pulse the eggplant flesh a few times. Add the garlic, onion, oregano, cumin, and lemon juice, and then gradually add the olive oil while the food processor is pulsing. Season with salt and freshly ground pepper and pulse. Transfer this mixture to a bowl and fold in the peppers. Let sit at room temperature for one hour before serving.

Spinach with Tangerine Dressing, Pancetta, Shallots, Gorgonzola, and Pine Nuts _____

Lombardi's, Dallas, TX

Chef: David Sonzugni

4 servings—690 calories per serving

> 1/4 cup olive oil
> 8 ounces pancetta, julienned
> 1/2 cup fresh shallots, sliced
> 2 cups tangerine or orange juice
> 1/2 cup champagne vinegar
> 1 cup fresh spinach, rinsed, stems trimmed
> 4 ounces gorgonzola cheese
> 1/4 cup pine nuts, toasted

In a large skillet over medium heat, add olive oil and pancetta. Brown pancetta evenly until crisp. Add shallots and cook until translucent. Add tangerine juice and champagne vinegar. Turn heat up to high. Reduce dressing until slightly thick. Place spinach on plates. Spoon dressing over spinach, making sure pancetta and shallots are distributed evenly. Sprinkle gorgonzola and pine nuts over the top and serve immediately.

Summer Bread Salad with Tomatoes, Cucumber, Basil, and Balsamic Vinaigrette _____

Higgins, Portland, OR

Chef: Greg Higgins

8 servings—214 calories per serving

> 1 loaf sourdough bread
> 1/2 cup olive oil

2 tablespoons garlic, minced

salt and freshly ground pepper to taste

1/4 cup balsamic vinegar

1 bunch basil

1 medium cucumber, peeled, seeded, and diced

2 large vine-ripened tomatoes, diced

1 head romaine lettuce, cleaned and dried

Preheat oven to 400 degrees. Slice four 1/2-inch slices of the bread and then dice the cut bread evenly. Toss the bread cubes with a drizzle of olive oil, 1 tablespoon garlic, and a pinch of salt and pepper. Toast them lightly over medium heat in a shallow pan until barely crisp, about 7 to 10 minutes. While the croutons are toasting, combine the remaining olive oil, garlic, and balsamic vinegar. Season to taste with salt and pepper. Set aside 4 basil tops for garnish. Slice the remaining basil into thin strips. Place the cucumbers and tomatoes in a bowl. Add the lightly toasted croutons, balsamic vinegar mixture, and the basil strips. Toss gently. Arrange the salad mixture on top of the leaves of romaine on four plates. Drizzle with the dressing from the bowl and garnish each with a basil sprig.

Note: Bay shrimp, cooked chicken breast, or cheese such as feta or ricotta salata may be added to create a more substantial meal.

Chicken, Fish, and Shellfish

Barcelona Stir Fry

Cafe Tu Tango, Ventura, FL

Chef: Monica Schatz

2 servings—380 calories per serving

1/4 cup olive oil

4 ounces boneless chicken, diced

4 ounces shrimp, peeled and deveined

4 ounces calamari rings, 1/2 inch thick

1 tablespoon garlic, chopped

6 ounces red, green, and yellow bell peppers, chopped

4 ounces mushrooms, sliced

4 ounces andouille sausage, diced

3/4 cup stir-fry sauce (mix together 1/4 cup each; lemon juice, chicken stock, and white wine)

1/2 teaspoon parsley, chopped

Heat oil in sauté pan over medium-high heat. Sauté chicken until cooked through, about 3 to 5 minutes. Add seafood and garlic. Continue to cook until shrimp is almost pink, about 3 minutes. Add peppers, mushrooms, and sausage, cooking until sausage is cooked through, about 5 minutes. Add stir-fry sauce and deglaze pan. Garnish with chopped parsley and serve.

Chicken Rouge

Christopher Martins, New Haven, CT
Chef: Mary Melie

2 servings—545 calories per serving

2 tablespoons extra-virgin olive oil

3/4 pound chicken tenders (or skinless, boneless breasts cut into strips)

4 tablespoons flour

1 tablespoon garlic, chopped

10 ounces wild mushrooms, sliced (mix of sliced portobello, shiitake, and oyster mushrooms, but button mushrooms can be substituted)

1 teaspoon fresh rosemary, chopped

6 ounces red wine

8 ounces chicken stock

salt and pepper to taste

1/2 pound linguini, cooked

Heat oil in a pan over medium heat. Dredge the chicken in flour and carefully place in pan. Cook for about 3 minutes. Turn chicken and add garlic. Cook for 1 minute. Push chicken to one side of pan. Add mushrooms, rosemary, red wine and stock, bring to a simmer, and reduce by half, about 10 minutes. Add salt and pepper to taste. Toss with warm linguini and serve immediately. (If using cold or precooked pasta, add it to the pan while the sauce is simmering and turn once before serving.)

Cod Braised with White Wine, Potatoes, and Escarole _____

The Blue Room, Cambridge, MA

Chef/owner: Steve Johnson

8 servings—485 calories per serving

1 pound salt cod, cut into small pieces and soaked overnight

1 Spanish onion, peeled and sliced

2 leeks, sliced and rinsed well

4 russet potatoes, peeled and cut into half-rounds

1 head escarole, rinsed well and chopped

4 garlic cloves, chopped

1 cup olive oil

2 cups white wine

1 teaspoon fresh thyme

2 quarts water

salt and pepper

lemon wedges

6 ounces fresh, boneless, skinless cod filet

Drain the salt cod. Place all ingredients except fresh cod into a large stockpot and simmer gently for about 90 minutes. The starch from the potatoes should just start to thicken the liquid.

Per serving: Heat 1 tablespoon of olive oil in a large sauté pan and sear one side of cod filet until golden in color. Flip the fish over and add about a 1/2 cup ladle of the salt cod and escarole stew to the skillet. When the liquid comes to a boil, cover and lower heat to medium low. Simmer the cod filet until it is just cooked through, about 4 to 5 minutes. Be careful not to let the liquid over-reduce— if this should happen, simply add a little water to the skillet to return the broth to its original consistency. Add salt or a squeeze of lemon to taste. Serve in individual bowls with a wedge of toasted focaccia or bread to soak up the broth.

Cuban-Style Braised Tuna* _____

White Dog Cafe, Philadelphia, PA

Chef: Keven von Klaus

Cuban cuisine is inherited from many cultures, including Ciboney Indian, African, Chinese, and Spanish. The most evident flavors are from Spain, which can be found in everything from saffron-infused rice dishes and flan to chorizo and olives and their oil. In this recipe, almonds, capers, and olives speak of the early Spaniards who brought the flavors of the Mediterranean to the islands of the Caribbean.

4 servings—550 calories per serving

1/4 cup extra-virgin olive oil

1 1/2 cups white onions, thinly sliced

2 tablespoons garlic, minced

4 cups fresh plum tomatoes, chopped

1/4 cup capers, rinsed and squeezed dry

1/3 cup pimento-stuffed green olives, sliced

pinch hot red pepper flakes

1 1/2 cups dry white wine

4 yellowfin tuna steaks (about 6 ounces each)

1/4 cup fresh cilantro, chopped

1/4 cup slivered almonds, toasted

Heat the oil in a large sauté pan or skillet over medium-high heat. Add the onions and cook until soft, about 4 minutes. Add the garlic and cook for 1 minute. Add the tomatoes and sauté until softened, about 3 minutes. Add the capers, olives, pepper flakes, and wine. Bring to a simmer. Add the tuna steaks. Reduce heat to low, cover, and simmer until the tuna is completely cooked through, 10 to 15 minutes, depending upon thickness of steaks. Remove the tuna and keep warm. If the sauce is too thin, increase the heat and simmer until it reduces to the desired consistency. Stir in the cilantro. Top the fish with the warm sauce and sprinkle with almonds. Serve with Lemon-Garlic Rice (see page 282).

From the White Dog Cafe Cookbook (Running Press, 1998)

Gazpacho Crab Cocktail _____

Baywolf Restaurant, Oakland, CA
Chef/owner: Michael Wild

2 servings—80 calories per serving

1 shallot, minced

1 teaspoon lemon juice

1/2 cup red bell pepper, diced

1/2 cup green bell pepper, diced

1/2 cup cucumber, peeled, seeded, and diced

2 ripe tomatoes, skinned and chopped

1 tablespoon chopped parsley

2 tablespoons celery, diced

1 tablespoon celery greens (the leaves of the heart), chopped

1/2 tablespoon Tabasco sauce

1/3 pound lump or flaked crabmeat, picked over
   salt and pepper to taste

Combine the minced shallot and lemon juice in a large bowl. Let sit for 15 minutes. Add the bell peppers, cucumber, tomatoes, parsley, celery, Tabasco sauce, and crabmeat. Season to taste with salt and pepper. Serve chilled.

Note: If tomatoes are not in season, canned, diced tomatoes can be substituted.

Lobster Fra Diavolo

Raphael Bar Risto, Providence, RI; East Greenwich, RI
Chef: Ralph Conte

1 serving—530 calories

1 lobster (1 1/2-pounds)

1/2 cup onions, sliced into thin strips

1/2 teaspoon nonpareil capers (nonpareils are the smaller of the two varieties commonly available and have the best flavor)

4 Sicilian olives

1 tablespoon extra-virgin olive oil

1 teaspoon crushed red pepper

3/4 cup white wine

1/2 cup fresh tomatoes, chopped, drained, and seeded

dash of fresh oregano, chopped

fresh basil, chopped

Boil the lobster. Remove meat from claws, knuckles, and tail. Reserve the head.

Combine onions, capers, olives, and olive oil in a large skillet over high heat and cook until onions become translucent. Add crushed red pepper and white wine and reduce heat to medium. Add chopped tomatoes and oregano and simmer for 3 minutes. Add lobster meat and lobster head and cook for 2 minutes. Serve over fettuccine, capellini, or linguine. Top with fresh basil.

Rainbow Trout with Cucumber Relish _____

Christopher Martins, New Haven, CT

Chef: Mary Melie

2 servings—650 calories per serving

3 tablespoons olive oil

2 12-ounce trout filets, heads and tails removed

3 tablespoons flour

salt and pepper to taste

Tomato, Basil, and Cucumber Relish (see page 292)

Heat pan over medium heat. Add oil. Flour trout and place fish in pan, flesh-side down. Cook for about 3 minutes or until the fish starts to turn white on edges. Carefully turn with spatula, so as not to break filets. Cook skin-side down for 3 minutes or until fish is firm and flaky to touch. Remove to plates and top with 2 tablespoons Tomato, Basil, and Cucumber Relish. Add salt and pepper to taste.

Seafood Caldo Verde

From Legal Sea Foods, Inc., Burlington, MA; Chestnut Hill, MA; Boston, MA; Prudential, MA; Cambridge, MA; Natick, MA; Peabody, MA; Nyack, NY; Warwick, RI; Washington, DC; McLean, VA

Executive chef: Richard Vellante

An adaptation of the classic Portuguese caldo verde, this dish is great on a cold autumn night as an appetizer or as a meal with a green salad.

4 servings—740 calories per serving

> 1 pound potatoes, peeled and sliced thin
> 1/2 cup extra-virgin olive oil
> 1 teaspoon salt
> 2 cloves garlic, peeled
> 1/2 cup dried pepperoncini, crumbled
> 4 sprigs fresh thyme
> 2 teaspoons olive oil
> 1 pound linguica or chorizo sausage, sliced 1/4-inch thick
> 8 littleneck clams, washed
> 1 pound mussels, washed
> 1/2 cup white wine
> 1/4 pound kale, thinly sliced

Place potatoes in a large soup pot with 3 cups of water and olive oil. Add salt, garlic, dried pepperoncini, and thyme and bring to boil. Reduce heat so soup boils gently. Whisk occasionally to break up potatoes. Cook until the potatoes completely dissolve and you have a shiny, lightly thickened broth, about 35 minutes.

Heat olive oil in a sauté pan. Add sausage and brown. Add shellfish and white wine, cover, and steam shellfish open, about 8 to 10 minutes. Add shellfish, sausage, and liquid soup. Add kale to soup and simmer for 2 minutes. Ladle soup into bowls and serve immediately with crusty bread.

Seafood Paella

Christopher Martins, New Haven, CT
Chef: Mary Melie

4 servings—694 calories per serving

> 2 tablespoons olive oil
> 1/2 pound turkey sausage (not breakfast style)
> 2 chicken breasts, halved
> 1 tablespoon chopped garlic
> 1 green pepper, seeded and diced
> 6 ounces roasted red peppers
> 1 cup white rice
> 1/2 cup white wine
> 2 cups shrimp stock
> 1 pound littleneck clams
> 1 pound mussels
> 1/2 pound large shrimp
> 1/2 pound scallops
> 1/2 pound whitefish such as scrod, cod, or haddock
> 1 tablespoon saffron
> 1 teaspoon tarragon
> 1 tablespoon oregano
> 1 tablespoon basil
> 1 teaspoon thyme
> 1/2 cup diced tomatoes

salt and pepper to taste

4 scallions, chopped

Heat the oil over medium heat in a large stockpot. Add the sausage and chicken and brown, 5 to 10 minutes. Stir in the garlic, peppers, and rice. Add the wine and stock and simmer 5 minutes. Add the seafood, fish, saffron, herbs, and tomatoes. Cover, reduce heat, and simmer for about 15 minutes or until shellfish open and rice is tender. Salt and pepper to taste and garnish with scallions. Season and serve with crusty bread.

Seared Tuna

Cafe Tu Tango, Ventura, FL
Chef: Monica Schatz

1 serving—160 calories

4 ounce tuna steak

1 teaspoon coarsely black pepper

1/2 teaspoon kosher salt

1 teaspoon white sesame seeds

Roll tuna in black pepper, salt, and sesame seeds. Quickly sear in a hot pan, and let cool. With sharp knife, slice tuna into 1-ounce medallions and serve.

Shrimp and Fennel

Christopher Martins, New Haven, CT
Chef: Mary Melie

2 servings—695 calories per serving

2 tablespoons extra-virgin olive oil

1 tablespoon chopped garlic

1/2 bulb fennel, cored and sliced crosswise

1/2 pound medium shrimp, peeled and deveined

4 ounces white wine

6 ounces fresh plum tomatoes, diced

1 ounce fresh basil, chopped

salt and pepper to taste

1/2 pound pasta such as spinach fettuccini, cooked

Heat skillet on medium heat. Add the oil, garlic, and fennel. Cook for about 4 to 5 minutes or until fennel starts to turn translucent. Add shrimp and let cook on one side for 90 seconds. Add wine. Turn shrimp and add the tomatoes and basil. Season with salt and pepper. Toss with warm pasta and enjoy.

Shrimp with Lemon-Date Dressing _____

by Patricia L. Wilson, Ph.D., Host of *What's Cooking with Patricia?* WOSO Radio, San Juan

8 servings—275 calories per serving

1 pound dates, pitted and chopped (fresh or dried)

juice of 1 lemon

1 cup fresh orange juice

1 tablespoon orange zest

1 bunch scallions, sliced

2 pounds tiny shrimp, steamed until just pink and cooled

orange sections for garnish

Place dates in large skillet, barely cover with water, and simmer for 5 minutes or until very tender. Mash the dates and mix with the lemon juice, orange juice, and orange zest (this can be done in a food processor). Mix the date dressing and the scallions with the cooled shrimp. Mound on a round platter and garnish with orange sections.

Swordfish with Three Sauces _____

Christopher Martins, New Haven, CT

Chef: Mary Melie

2 servings—500 calories per serving

> 1 cup pine nuts
> salt and pepper to taste
> 1/4 cup flour
> 2 6-ounce swordfish (or tuna) steaks
> 1/2 cup 1%-low-fat milk
> olive oil
> Tapenade (see page 289)
> Basil Pesto (see. page 286)
> Sun-Dried Tomato Pesto (see page 289)

Place the pine nuts in a food processor and process to almost a fine powder. Add salt and pepper and combine with flour. Soak fish in milk and dredge in pine-nut flour mixture. In a large sauté pan on medium heat, add just enough olive oil to cover the bottom of the pan. Add the fish and cook on one side. Turn over and finish to desired doneness (i.e., rare to medium rare for tuna or medium for swordfish). Fish takes 10 minutes total cooking time per inch of thickness. Top with one stripe each of Tapenade (see page 289), Basil Pesto (page 286), and Sun-Dried Tomato Pesto (page 289).

Vegetables and Accompaniments

Eggplant Caponata _____

The University Club, Providence, RI
Chef: Gary Camella

12 1/2-cup-servings—110 calories per serving

>   2 pounds eggplant, peeled and cut into 1 inch cubes
>   salt
>   1 large onion, coarsely chopped
>   1/4 cup olive oil
>   1 cup Salsa di Pomodoro Passata (see page 288)
>   1/2 cup tomato paste
>   1 stalk celery, strings removed and coarsely chopped
>   6 tablespoons white raisins
>   3/4 to 1 cup green olives, pitted and cut into thirds
>   4 tablespoons capers, rinsed and drained
>   3 tablespoons sugar
>   1/2 cup red wine vinegar
>   black pepper
>   olive oil for frying
>   chopped basil
>   chopped parsley

Place eggplant cubes in a colander and salt them. Let stand for 1 hour. Heat olive oil in large pan over medium heat and sauté onions until just golden, about 2 to 3 minutes. Add salsa di pomodoro passata and tomato paste. Simmer uncovered until thickened, 5 to 8 minutes. Add celery, raisins, olives, capers, sugar, vinegar, and salt and pepper to taste. Simmer for 15 to 20 minutes, then transfer sauce to a large bowl and cool. Heat 1 inch of oil in a large sauté pan. Wipe eggplant pieces dry, and fry them a batch at a time, until golden brown. Drain well on paper towels. Add the eggplant to the sauce and mix well. Taste for seasoning. Sprinkle with parsley and basil and serve at room temperature.

Esparragos a La Navarra

Emilio's Tapas Chicago, Chicago, IL
Chef/Owner: Emilio Gervilla

2 to 3 servings—88 calories per 2 servings

> 3 white asparagus spears
> 1/2 yellow tomato, sliced
> 1/3 roasted red pepper, sliced
> 2 teaspoons sherry vinegar
> 1/8 cup Pedro Ximenez sherry (fino)

Place the asparagus spears on a plate with the points coming together in the middle. Arrange tomatoes in between asparagus and place the roasted peppers on top. Mix together the vinegar and sherry and pour over.

Grilled Portobello Mushrooms with Escarole and Pine Nuts

Christopher Martins, New Haven, CT
Chef: Mary Melie

These "meaty" mushrooms pick up their best flavor from the grill, but you can roast them in the oven with similar results.

2 servings—480 calories per serving

> 2 large portobello mushrooms, stems removed
> 3 tablespoons extra-virgin olive oil

2 tablespoons garlic, chopped

1/4 cup pine nuts, toasted

1/2 cup Marsala wine

1 large head escarole, washed and chopped

salt and pepper to taste

Brush mushroom caps with 1 tablespoon oil on underside only and place on preheated grill or broiler. Cook over medium heat for 4 to 5 minutes or until the mushrooms start to soften. Turn over and grill for another 4 minutes. Set aside. Place remaining oil and garlic in medium pan over medium heat. Cook until just brown. Add nuts and wine. Cook until the liquid is reduced by half. Add escarole and cook until wilted. Season with salt and pepper. Top with cooked mushroom caps and serve.

Grilled Vegetables Provencal Style _____

Christopher Martins, New Haven, CT

Chef: Mary Melie

6 servings—150 calories per serving

1 medium zucchini, trimmed and halved lengthwise

1 medium yellow squash, trimmed and halved lengthwise

1 red or yellow pepper, seeded and sliced

1 green pepper, seeded and sliced

1 small eggplant, trimmed and halved lengthwise

4 ounces button mushrooms, halved

1 medium red onion, peeled and halved lengthwise

3/4 cup extra-virgin olive oil

3 tablespoons chopped garlic

salt and pepper to taste

1/4 cup fresh basil leaves, chopped

2 tablespoons fresh rosemary, chopped

2 tablespoons fresh sage, chopped

6 tablespoons balsamic vinegar

Preheat grill to medium high. Place zucchini, squash, peppers, eggplants, mushrooms, and onion in a large bowl and toss with the garlic and 4 ounces of oil. Season with salt and pepper. Place zucchini, squash, onion, and eggplant on lower rack and peppers and mushrooms on higher rack to prevent burning. Cook until just tender, turning once. Remove to bowl. Add the herbs, the remaining oil, and the vinegar. Let stand 30 minutes, tossing once. Serve with greens or grilled items and sliced tomatoes.

Grilled Vegetables Tenerife

From The Spanish Tavern Restaurant, Narragansett, RI

Chefs: Guilleromo Vasconcelos and Jose Da Silva

Grilling gives fresh vegetables a distinct and delicious flavor. It is a fast and easy cooking method; however, cooking times will vary depending on the ripeness and size of the vegetables. Avoid overcooking by checking for readiness after ten minutes—this will also allow the vegetables to be nice and moist. Enjoy!

2 servings—175 calories per serving

4 whole, fresh asparagus

4 large, fresh mushrooms

3 or 4 sweet red peppers, cut in 1-inch slices

1 large onion, sliced

3 or 4 green and yellow squash, cut in 3/4-inch pieces

2 tablespoons olive oil

2 tablespoons balsamic vinegar or red wine vinegar

1/2 teaspoon dried basil or oregano

Heat the grill over medium heat. Arrange the asparagus, mushrooms, peppers, onion, and squash on the grill, making sure they are not directly on the flame, about 5 inches away. Mix the olive oil, balsamic vinegar, basil or oregano and occasionally brush the vegetables to prevent them from drying out.

Variation: Marinate the vegetables in the olive oil/balsamic vinegar mixture for about 10 minutes before grilling.

Imam Baildi

Taverna Cretekou, Alexandria, VA

Chef: George Maltabes

12 servings—260 calories per serving

12 small baby eggplants, about 2 pounds

1 1/4 cup olive oil

salt to taste

4 cups onions, sliced

2 tablespoons garlic, peeled and minced

1/2 cup parsley, chopped

1 stick cinnamon

2 pieces clove

3 large tomatoes, peeled, seeded, and chopped, or 2
    cups crushed tomatoes

1/2 cup water

1/2 teaspoon salt

1/4 teaspoon pepper

2 tablespoons pine nuts

2 tablespoons white raisins

Preheat oven to 350 degrees. Cut two lengthwise slits along each eggplant. Brush on all sides with 1/4 cup olive oil and salt lightly. Place in a baking dish and bake for 20 minutes or until soft. In a large pan over medium heat, sauté onions and garlic in remaining cup of olive oil until soft. Add parsley, tomatoes, water, cinnamon, cloves, pine nuts, raisins, salt, and pepper. Bring to a boil and simmer for 15 minutes. Carefully spoon some sauce into the incisions in the eggplants. Pour remaining sauce over eggplants and continue to bake for 10 minutes. Serve at room temperature.

Lemon-Garlic Rice* _____

White Dog Cafe, Philadelphia, PA
Chef: Kevin von Klaus

2 servings—185 calories per serving

> 2 tablespoons olive oil
> 1/2 cup white onion, minced
> 2 tablespoons garlic, minced
> 1 cup long-grain white rice, uncooked
> 2 cups water
> salt
> juice of 1/2 lemon
> grated or minced zest of 1 whole lemon
> freshly ground black pepper

Heat oil in a saucepan over medium high heat. Add the onion and cook until soft, about 5 minutes. Add the garlic and cook for 1 minute. Add the rice and toss to coat with the oil. Pour in the water, a pinch of salt, and lemon juice. Bring to a boil. Cover and reduce the heat to low. Simmer until the rice is cooked and the

_____
From the White Dog Cafe Cookbook (Running Press, 1998)

liquid is absorbed, 20 to 25 minutes. Remove from heat and fluff with a fork. Toss with the lemon zest, season to taste with salt and pepper, and serve immediately.

Marsini's Black-Eyed Peas

Tosca, Hingham, MA
Chef: Joe Simone

8 servings—85 calories per serving

> 2 cups cold water
> dash of salt
> 4 cups black-eyed peas
> 1/4 cup extra-virgin olive oil
> 1 1/2 cups onion, finely diced
> 1 1/2 cups green onions or young leeks, finely chopped
> 5 cups loosely packed fennel tops
> 2 cups tomato concasse
> salt and pepper to taste

Bring a large pot of salted water to boil. Parboil the black-eyed peas 10 minutes or until al dente. Drain the black-eyed peas well. In a large saucepan, heat the oil and add onion and leeks. When onion is tender, add the fennel tops and stir for 1 minute. Add cold water and stir to combine. Simmer for 10 minutes until liquid is reduced and the vegetables are tender. Add tomato concasse and cook for 1 minute. Add beans and simmer until tender, about 20 minutes. Add salt and pepper to taste and serve.

Note: To prepare fennel tops, choose young, fragrant greens. Remove the tough stems and wash. Cut into 1-inch pieces.

Plato Sorpresa

Emilio's Tapas Chicago, Chicago, IL
Chef/Owner: Emilio Gervilla

2 to 3 servings—370 calories per 2 servings

>   3 tablespoons extra-virgin olive oil
>   1 ball fresh mozzarella, cut in 1/4-pieces
>   1/2 red tomato, sliced
>   1/2 yellow tomato, sliced
>   1/4 red onion, thinly sliced
>   5 Kalamata olives, sliced
>   fresh basil, chopped
>   salt and pepper to taste

Pour the olive oil in a pool on the bottom of a plate. Alternate pieces of mozzarella, tomatoes, and onions on top. Place the olives and basil on top. Add salt and pepper to taste and serve.

Risotto Cakes

Christopher Martins, New Haven, CT
Chef: Mary Melie
Risotto is as versatile as pasta, but requires a little patience.
4 servings—312 calories per serving

>   2 1/2 cups chicken stock, boiling
>   3 tablespoons extra-virgin olive oil
>   1/2 cup onion, finely diced
>   1 cup arborio rice
>   salt and pepper to taste
>   4 ounces Parmesan cheese
>   1/2 cup flour

1/2 teaspoon garlic, chopped

1 cup wild mushrooms, sliced

1 teaspoon fresh basil, chopped

3 ounces dry white wine

Bring chicken stock to a boil in a medium saucepan, then reduce heat to simmer. Heat 2 tablespoons of oil in a large saucepan over low heat. Add onion and cook until the onion is translucent. Add the rice and stir with a nonmetal spoon until the rice starts to turn translucent, about 8 minutes. Increase the heat to medium low. Add the hot stock 1/2 cup at a time, stirring constantly with spoon. Do not add more stock until the previous batch has been absorbed. This method allows the rice to become creamy as the starch is released into the liquid. Continue adding stock until all is absorbed. The rice grains should be just cooked, with a very slight crunch to them. Season with salt and pepper. Add 3 ounces of cheese, stirring until incorporated.

Cool risotto in a pan greased with olive oil, uncovered, for two hours, then form risotto into patties using about 1/2 cup of rice for each. Lightly dredge each risotto cake with flour. Heat 1 tablespoon olive oil in a medium-sized pan over medium heat. Brown both sides of the risotto cake, remove to a plate, and keep warm. Add garlic, mushrooms, and basil to the pan and stir. Add wine and deglaze pan. Pour over risotto cake and top with the remaining cheese. Serve over marinara sauce or fresh roasted tomato sauce.

Roasted Garlic

Christopher Martins, New Haven, CT

Chef: Mary Melie

3 garlic bulbs

1/2 cup olive oil

Peel garlic cloves completely. Place garlic and oil in small pan so that garlic is in single layer on bottom of pan and oil just covers cloves. Heat on high heat until oil starts to boil. Gently turn cloves with spoon to cook evenly. When browning starts, remove from heat and cool. Roasted garlic can be stored in the refrigerator for up to 2 weeks in oil. The oil also can be used to flavor other dishes.

Roasted Peppers

Christopher Martins, New Haven, CT
Chef: Mary Melie

5 pounds red bell peppers
paper bag

Preheat oven to 500 degrees. Place peppers in a roasting pan in a single layer. Cook, turning once, for about 20 minutes or until skins are black and puffy. Carefully place peppers into a paper bag and seal. Remove peppers from bag after 20 minutes (the skins should slide off easily). Remove stems and seeds. Roasted peppers can be stored in the refrigerator for up to 1 week or frozen for 1 month in small batches.

Tabbouleh

Christopher Martins, New Haven
Chef: Mary Melie

Tabbouleh is Middle Eastern in origin and can be used as a main dish or an accompaniment.

8 servings—133 calories per serving

3/4 cup bulgur wheat

1 3/4 cups hot water

1/2 cup fresh parsley, chopped

1/4 cup fresh mint, chopped

3/4 cup lemon juice

4 medium plum tomatoes, finely chopped

6 tablespoons olive oil

salt and pepper to taste

In a covered pan, steep the bulgur wheat in hot water about 15 minutes. Uncover and let cool 10 minutes. Add the herbs, lemon juice, tomatoes, and oil. Cover loosely and refrigerate for 1 hour. Serve with grilled fish, chicken, or pork.

Vegetable Penne

Christopher Martins, New Haven, CT

Chef: Mary Melie

2 servings—525 calories per serving

1 tablespoon olive oil

1 tablespoon garlic, chopped

1/2 teaspoon red pepper flakes

1/4 cup leeks, sliced thin

1/4 cup sliced mushrooms

1/3 cup roasted red peppers

2 tablespoons fresh oregano, chopped

2 carrots, sliced thin

1 head broccoli cut into florets

1 small zucchini, sliced

1 small yellow squash, sliced

salt and pepper to taste

1/3 cup dry white wine

3/4 cup chicken stock

8 ounces cooked penne pasta

1/4 cup Parmesan cheese, grated

Heat oil in large sauté pan over medium heat. Add garlic, pepper flakes, leeks, mushrooms, and peppers. Stir occasionally until the leeks are translucent and the mushrooms are cooked through, about 3 minutes. Add oregano, carrots, broccoli, zucchini, and squash. Season with salt and pepper. Cook 2 minutes. Add wine and stock and deglaze pan. Toss with cooked penne and vegetables. Sprinkle with cheese and serve.

Sauces and Toppings

Basil Pesto

Christopher Martins, New Haven, CT
Chef: Mary Melie

19 tablespoon-servings—70 calories per tablespoon

1 cup packed, fresh basil

1/3 cup pine nuts

1/4 cup grated Parmesan cheese

1 ounce dry white wine

1/2 cup extra-virgin olive oil

Purée the first three ingredients in a food processor. Add the wine and oil and process until smooth. Can be made in advance and kept for 2 weeks in the refrigerator or can be frozen for up to 1 month.

Marinara Sauce

Christopher Martins, New Haven, CT
Chef: Mary Melie

8 1/2-cup-servings—120 calories per serving

>   3 tablespoons olive oil
>   1 small onion, diced
>   1 teaspoon rosemary
>   1 teaspoon thyme
>   1 cup white wine
>   2 28-ounce cans whole tomatoes, drained (reserve liquid)
>   salt and pepper to taste
>   1/2 cup garlic, roasted (see page 283)
>   1/4 cup fresh parsley, chopped

Heat oil over in large pot over medium heat. Add onion and herbs and cook until onion is translucent, 3 to 5 minutes. Add wine and reduce liquid to half. In a large bowl, gently crush the tomatoes with a spoon. Add tomatoes to pot and bring to a boil.

Reduce heat and simmer for three hours. Season with salt and pepper. Add roasted garlic and parsley. Can be made ahead and refrigerated up to 1 week or frozen up to 1 month in single-serving containers.

Puttanesca Sauce

Christopher Martins, New Haven, CT
Chef: Mary Melie

2 servings—635 calories per serving

>   1 tablespoon olive oil
>   1 tablespoon garlic, chopped

1 ounce canned anchovy filets, chopped

2 tablespoons capers (nonpareils)

2/3 cup Kalamata olives, pitted and sliced

1/4 cup dry white wine

12 ounces marinara sauce (see page 287)

2 tablespoons parsley, chopped

2 tablespoons fresh basil, chopped

12 ounces cooked linguini

Heat oil in medium pan on medium-high heat. Add garlic and anchovies. Reduce heat to medium. As garlic begins to brown and anchovies start to break up, 2 to 3 minutes, add the capers and olives. Add wine, deglaze, and reduce fluid by half. Add marinara sauce and herbs. Toss with cooked pasta. Serve with crusty bread and Parmesan cheese.

Salsa di Pomodoro Passata
(Smooth Tomato Paste)

The University Club, Providence, RI
Chef: Gary Camella

3 1-cup servings—210 calories per serving

2 pounds Italian plum tomatoes (use fresh when in season)

1 large onion, finely chopped

2 garlic cloves, peeled and minced

1/4 cup olive oil

1 teaspoon sugar

1/4 cup basil leaves

salt

black pepper

If using fresh tomatoes, peel and halve them and place in medium pan over medium heat. Cover, cook until soft, and pass through a food mill. If using canned tomatoes, blend in a food processor and reserve in bowl. Heat the olive oil in a medium pot over medium heat and sauté the onion and garlic until golden, about 2 to 3 minutes. Add the tomato purée, sugar, basil, and salt and pepper to taste. Cook for at least 20 minutes or until the sauce is reduced and thickened to your liking.

Sun-Dried Tomato Pesto

Christopher Martins, New Haven, CT
Chef: Mary Melie

18 tablespoon-servings—80 calories per tablespoon

> 3/4 cup sun-dried tomatoes, soaked in oil or water and
> drained (save liquid)
> 1/3 cup pine nuts
> 1/4 cup grated Parmesan cheese
> 1/2 cup oil from the sun-dried tomatoes or extra-virgin
> olive oil

Purée the first 3 ingredients, adding oil slowly. Can be made in advance and kept for 2 weeks in the refrigerator or can be frozen and reheated.

Tappenade

Christopher Martins, New Haven, CT
Chef: Mary Melie

19 tablespoon-servings—60 calories per tablespoon

> 1/2 cup Kalamata olives, pitted

2 tablespoons garlic, roasted (see recipe on page 283)

1 tablespoon anchovies

1 tablespoon fresh basil

about 1/2 cup extra-virgin olive oil

Combine first 4 ingredients in food processor and pulse until chopped fine. Slowly add oil and process until smooth. Can be made in advance and kept for 2 weeks in the refrigerator.

Tomato, Basil, and Cucumber Relish

Christopher Martins, New Haven, CT
Chef: Mary Melie

22 tablespoon-servings—20 calories per tablespoon

1 medium red onion, diced small

1 medium cucumber, peeled, seeded, and diced small

3 plum tomatoes (about 6 ounces), diced small

1 teaspoon garlic, minced

3 tablespoons fresh basil, chopped

3 tablespoons extra-virgin olive oil

1/4 cup balsamic vinegar

salt and pepper to taste

Combine all ingredients in a small, nonmetal bowl. Let stand at room temperature for 30 minutes. Can be refrigerated for 1 week.

20 The Mediterranean Alternative Medicine Chest

By now you should realize the reason Mediterraneans live longer and healthier lives is not just because of the long walks, the sunny weather, and lower stress. It's the food and the phytochemicals, too. Phytochemicals help plants ward off infestation, fight infection and disease, resist oxidation, and protect against the DNA-damaging rays of the sun. These chemicals are the drugs that make up the Mediterranean Diet's Alternative Medicine Chest. Vegetable, fruits, nuts, and legumes together with the olive oil and red wine in the Mediterranean Diet contain a pharmacopoeia of compounds that would dwarf the inventory of any modern pharmacy and that can help protect us from diease. To give you an example of what's in fruits and vegetables we'll present some of the known phytochemicals in broccoli. After you read what's in this stuff you may want to bathe in it. It may even convince George Bush to eat some.

Broccoli

Broccoli is thought to have been developed by the ancient Romans or the Etruscans from the cabbage. Hence like cabbage, brussels sprouts, cauliflower, and arugula, broccoli is a cruciferous vegetable. Here's what's in it:

beta-carotene. This is only one of hundreds of carotenoids, but it is by far the most famous. It was among the first phytochemicals we discovered and could measure in the blood. Beta-carotene is a potent antioxidant and is particularly effective at soothing dangerous, oxidized oxygen molecules. (Beta-carotene is also found in carrots.)

benzyl isothiocyanate. Benzyl isothiocyanate can not only prevent the formation of some carcinogens including the lung carcinogens in tobacco smoke, it can even suppress tumor growth in cells already damaged by carcinogens. Benzyl isothiocyanate can also suppress the formation of heterocyclic amines that are created when meat is seared brown.

beta-ionone. This is produced when beta-carotene quenches oxygen free radicals. It not only neutralizes the cancer-causing potential of certain carcinogens, but it also prevents cancer cells from multiplying by inhibiting an enzyme critical to cell growth.

carotenoids. These are a group of compounds. More than five hundred carotenoids have been discovered, but scientists have studied only about fifty of them. Some of the carotenoids are beta- and alpha-carotene, lutein, and lycopene. Best known for being antioxidants, carotenoids have a variety of health-promoting functions. Carotenoids need fat to be absorbed. (Carotenoids are also found in apricots, basil, bay leaves, carrots, peppers, and spinach.)

coumarin. Coumarin can induce an enzyme that can detoxify cancer-causing compounds. Coumarin has also been shown to inhibit tumor growth in animals. (Coumarin is also found in lemons, oranges, and grapefruits.)

flavonoids. Flavonoids are another large group of phytochemicals that are potent antioxidants. Several large human population studies have related flavonoid intake to reduced incidence of heart attacks. Flavonoids also seem to stop tumors from growing in animals and to inhibit the activity of cyclooxygenase, leading to platelet aggregation and reducing the platelets' tendency to clot. Broccoli is known to carry many different flavonoids. (Flavonoids are also found in apples, red grapes, red wine, and onions.)

glucobrassin. One of the glucosinolates, glucobrassin has been shown to inhibit the induction of cancer cells in animals by promoting the activity of certain liver-based enzymes.

hydroxycinnamic acids. A group of flavonoids, these are highly effective in preventing lipid oxidation.

indole-3-carbinol. This is one of the glucosinolates. It is made from glucobrassin (another phytochemical) when the plant material is disrupted, such as by chewing or during food preparation. In rats, indole-3-carbinol has been shown to prevent the formation of a hormone-like compound that can potentially cause cancer. In animals, indole-3-carbinol also seems to help certain liver enzymes fight cancer. (Indole-3-carbinol is also found in leafy greens and other cruciferous vegetables such as brussels sprouts, cabbage, and cauliflower.)

isothiocyanates. These are flavonoids and may help prevent cancer at various stages. For instance, they inhibit DNA damage and the growth of cancerous cells once formed. In rats, they have been shown to blunt the carcinogenic effect of cigarette smoke and charred meat. Isothiocyanates can induce cancer-fighting enzymes. They also induce apoptosis, which is the body's mechanism for removing damaged or abnormal cells. (Isothiocyanates are also found in cruciferous vegetables such as brussels sprouts, cabbage, and cauliflower.)

kaemperol. Kaemperol is linked with one of the flavonoids associated with lower mortality from heart disease in humans. It is a potent antioxidant that has been shown to inhibit cell damage of oxygen free radicals in hamsters. It can also relax and dilate the blood vessels of rats. In a test tube, kaemperol can be converted into an estrogen-like compound that prevents hormone-dependent cancers in animals. It also has anti-inflammatory properties. Its antithyroid activity could play a role in preventing thyroid cancer. Finally, kaemperol inhibits platelet aggregation in ways similar to aspirin, thus discouraging clogged arteries.

phenethyl isothiocyanate. This is one of the most effective cancer chemopreventive phytochemicals known. Phenethyl isothiocyanate can induce apoptosis, a process by which the body removes abnormal cells without leaving any scar tissue. In a test tube, it inhibits tobacco byproducts from causing cancer. In rodents, it inhibits chemically induced breast, esophageal, gastrointestinal tract, and lung cancer formations. In rats, it induces a cancer-fighting enzyme in the esophagus and colon. (Phenethyl isothiocyanate is also found in cruciferous vegetables such as brussels sprouts, cabbage, and cauliflower.)

protease inhibitors. All the benefits of protease inhibitors are still unclear, but from laboratory experiments they seem to suppress cancerous changes in cells exposed to carcinogenic agents, and have inhibited tumors in laboratory animals. (Protease inhibitors are also found in chick peas, kidney beans, and spinach.)

quercetin. This is another flavonoid associated with lower human mortality from coronary heart disease. In a test tube, quercetin is a scavenger of oxygen's free radicals, thus inhibiting LDL oxidation and preventing free-radical chain reactions in cell membranes. Quercetin extends the life of vitamin C and has also been shown to inhibit blood clotting. In rabbits, quercetin preserves the level of nitric oxide in injured heart tissue and has anti-inflammatory effects. In mice, quercetin reduces the uptake of LDL by cells in blood vessel walls. It also inhibits the growth of cancer cells in animals. (Quercetin is also found in grapes, leafy greens, onions, potatoes, and tomatoes.)

sulforaphane. A flavonoid, it is a potent stimulator of the enzyme glutathione S-transferase (GST), which detoxifies potential carcinogens. In rats, sulforaphane reduces the incidence, number, size, and rate of development of mammary tumors. Sulforaphane is in broccoli itself, but much higher levels are found in broccoli sprouts.

terpenoids. Like polyphenols and carotenoids, terpenoids are a general group of phytochemicals. Terpenoids can work as antioxidants, which may inhibit the development of cancer and heart disease. They also seem to inhibit tumor growth even after abnormal cells have been activated. In laboratory animals terpenoids have lowered LDL cholesterol and stimulated enzyme GST that detoxifies potential carcinogens.

Pretty impressive. And that's just broccoli. How about artichokes, arugala, asparagus, spinach, escarole, kale, garlic, onions, eggplant, basil, tomatoes, peas, olives, grapes, lemons, tangerines, oranges, apples, strawberries, peppers, plums, and scores of other fruits and vegetables. There are literally tens of thousands of phytochemicals in these foods. Below we have listed about forty of the more well studied phytochemicals in the Mediterranean Diet and a brief description of one or two of their more well documented properties. (Most of this is from very recent research done in animals and test tubes.)

allyl sulfide	inhibits blood clotting
anthocyanin	antioxidant and inhibits blood clotting
caffeic acid	antioxidant, inhibits the development of cancerous cells; antibacterial and anti fungal
carnosol acid	antioxidant; stops tumors from growing
carvone	inhibits the development of cancerous cells
catechin	antioxidant and inhibits blood clotting
chlorogenic acid	antioxidant, inhibits the development of cancerous cells
chrysin	antioxidant and inhibits blood clotting
cinnamic acid	inhibits the development of cancerous cells
dithiolthiones	inhibits the development of cancerous cells
ellagic acid	inhibits the development of cancerous cells
epicatechin	antioxidant
eugenol	inhibits the development of cancerous cells
ferulic acid	antioxidant; inhibits the development of cancerous cells
fisetin	antioxidant and inhibits blood clotting

geraniol	inhibits the development of cancerous cells
glucarates	inhibits the development of cancerous cells
hydroxytyrosol	antioxidant and inhibits blood clotting
isoprenoids	inhibits the development of cancerous cells
leucocyanidol	anti-inflammatory; antioxidant
limonene	inhibits the development of cancerous cells
lutein	helps prevent age-related macular degeneration (blindness)
lycopene	potent antioxidant; inhibits the development of cancerous cells
myricetin	antioxidant and inhibits blood clotting
nobiletin	inhibits the development of cancerous cells; in rats, protects against ulcers
oleuropein	antioxidant; inhibits bacterial growth
perillyl alcohol	inhibits the development of cancerous cells
p-coumaric acid	inhibits the development of cancerous cells
polydatin	inhibits blood clotting
resveratrol	antioxidant and inhibits blood clotting
rutin	antioxidant; inhibits uric acid formation, so may help prevent gout
salicylic acid	anti-inflammatory; inhibits blood clotting
silymarin	antioxidant; inhibits the development of cancerous cells
squalene	inhibits the development of cancerous cells
tangeretin	inhibits the development of cancerous cells
tannic acid	inhibits the development of cancerous cells; antioxidant; promotes dilation of blood vessels through nitric oxide

taxifolin	antioxidant
ursolic acid	antioxidant; inhibits the development of cancerous cells

Of course a laundry list of chemicals is not too interesting and not at all appetizing. Frankly a long list of vegetables is not all that interesting or appetizing either. But add a little olive oil and suddenly you go from a mere collection of phytochemicals and vegetables to a cuisine—a remarkably simple, delicious, healthy and harmonious cuisine. The Mediterranean cuisine.

References

Page

Chapter One: A Matter of Life and Death

7. *The percentage of fat in the American diet has dropped by almost 15 percent...* Stephen AM, Wald NJ. Trends in individual consumption of dietary fat in the United States, 1920-1984. *Am J Clin Nutr* 1990; 52:457-469.

7. *And all this time, Americans have continued to get fatter.* Kuczmarski RJ, Flegal KM, Campbell SM, Johnson CL. Increasing prevalence of overweight among US adults. The National Health and Nutrition Examination Surveys, 1960 to 1991 [see comments]. *JAMA* 1994; 272:205-11.

7. *Very low-fat diets may even deprive the body...* Williams AW, Boileau TW, Erdman JW, Jr. Factors influencing the uptake and absorption of carotenoids. *Proc Soc Exp Biol Med* 1998; 218:106-8.

7. *And there is compelling new evidence that sometimes they can be positively unhealthy.* Krauss RM, Dreon DM. Low-density-lipoprotein subclasses and response to a low-fat diet in healthy men. *Am J Clin Nutr* 1995; 62:478S-487S.

7. *The no-fat/low-fat message has become so pervasive that in a poll...*

Schwartz NE, Borra ST. What do consumers really think about dietary fat? *J Am Diet Assoc* 1997; 97:S73-75.

Chapter 2: Why Low-Fat Diets Don't Work

20. *The American Heart Association diet guidelines have called...*Chait A, Brunzell JD, Denke MA, et al. Rationale of the diet-heart statement of the American Heart Association. Report of the Nutrition Committee [see comments]. *Circulation* 1993; 88:3008-29.

20. *For years the government's National Cholesterol Education Program...* National Cholesterol Education Program. Second Report of the Expert Panel on Detection, Evaluation, and Treatment of High Blood Cholesterol in Adults (Adult Treatment Panel II). *Circulation* 1994; 89:1333-445.

23. *For instance, if you tell human volunteers that one yogurt is low in fat...* Shide DJ, Rolls BJ. Information about the fat content of preloads influences energy intake in healthy women. *J Am Diet Assoc* 1995; 95:993-98.

23. *Other experiments show that people who think...* Rolls BJ, Miller DL. Is the low-fat message giving people a license to eat more? *J Am Coll Nutr* 1997; 16:535-43.

23. *In America, the biggest source of fat is the fat hidden in ground meat.* Block G, Dresser CM, Hartman AM, Carroll MD. Nutrient sources in the American diet: Quantitative data from the NHANES II Study. *Am J of Epidemiol* 1985; 122:27-40.

23. *Research shows that foods with high energy density like chocolate...* Drewnowski A. Why do we like fat? *J Am Diet Assoc* 1997; 97:S58-62.

24. *For instance, carbohydrates and especially fiber...* Rolls BJ. Carbohydrates, fats, and satiety. *Am J Clin Nutr* 1995; 61:960S-67S.

24. *The effects of fat on feeling full tend to show up after a few hours...* Sepple CP, Read NW. Effect of prefeeding lipid on food intake and satiety in man. Gut 1990; 31:158-61; Himaya A, Fantino M, Antoine JM, Brondel L, Louis-Sylvestre J. Satiety power of dietary fat: a new appraisal. *Am J Clin Nutr* 1997; 65:1410-18.

25. *Eating fat stimulates the release of hormones... Perspectives in Nutrition.* Wardlaw GM, Insel PM, eds. Boston, Massachusetts: WCB McGraw-Hill, 1996.

25. *The small intestine also has fat receptors...* Read N, French S, Cunningham K. The role of the gut in regulating food intake in man. *Nutr Rev* 1994; 52:1-10.

25. *Palatability (good taste) and satiety (feeling full)...* Drewnowski A. Energy density, palatability, and satiety: implications for weight control. *Nutr Rev* 1998; 56:347- 53.

25. *We asked physicians to tell us how many grams of fat...*Vigilante K, Flynn M. Inadequate physician knowledge of the effect of diet on blood lipids. *Circulation* 1998; 98:3075

26. *Researchers from Canada showed that animals...* Brooks S, Lampi B. Time course of enzyme changes after a switch from a high-fat to a low-fat diet. *Comp Biochem Physiol B Biochem Mol Biol* 1997; 118:359-65.

26. *Researchers from the Rockefeller University showed...* Hudgins LC, Hellerstein M, Seidman C, Neese R, Diakun J, Hirsch J. Human fatty acid synthesis is stimulated by a eucaloric low fat, high carbohydrate diet. *J Clin Invest* 1996; 97:2081-91.

26. *Researchers from the University of Colorado showed...* Yost TJ, Jensen DR, Haugen BR, Eckel RH. Effect of dietary macronutrient composition on tissue-specific lipoprotein lipase activity and insulin action in normal-weight subjects. *Am J Clin Nutr* 1998; 68:296-302.

27. *A researcher named Lauren Lissner did just that...* Lissner L, Heitmann BL. Dietary fat and obesity: evidence from epidemiology. *Eur J Clin Nutr* 1995; 49:79-90.

28. *Drs. Chen Junshi and Colin Campbell took a similar...* Chen J, Campbell T, Tunyao L, Peto R. *Diet, lifestyle and mortality in China: a study of the characteristics of 65 chinese countries.* Oxford: Oxford University Press, 1990.

28. *Some, but not all, short-term studies do show that....* Willett WC. Is dietary fat a major determinant of body fat? *Am J Clin Nutr* 1998; 67:556S-562S.

29. *For instance in another study by Dr. Lissner...* Lissner L, Levitsky DA, Strupp BJ, Kalkwarf HJ, Roe DA. Dietary fat and the regulation of energy intake in human subjects. *Am J Clin Nutr* 1987; 46:886-92.

29. *Coauthor Mary Flynn did an experiment...* Flynn MM, Zmuda JM, Milosavljevic D, Caldwell MJ, Herbert PN. Lipoprotein response to a National Cholesterol Education Program Step II Diet with and without energy restriction. *Metabolism* 1999; (in press).

31. *In the National Diet Heart Diet Study...* The National Diet-Heart Study Final Report. *Circulation.* 1968; 37:I1-428.

31. *The frequent failure of very-low-fat diets is well illustrated...* Knopp RH, Walden CE, Retzlaff BM, et al. Long-term cholesterol-lowering effects of 4 fat-restricted diets in hypercholesterolemic and com-

bined hyperlipidemic men. The Dietary Alternatives Study. *JAMA* 1997; 278:1509-15.

31.   *In 1998, Walter Willett, Chairman of Nutrition...* Willett WC. Is dietary fat a major determinant of body fat? *Am J Clin Nutr* 1998; 67:556S-62S.

Note: Some of the long-term studies he reviews are:

Kasim SE, Martino S, Kim PN, et al. Dietary and anthropometric determinants of plasma lipoproteins during a long-term low-fat diet in healthy women. *Am J Clin Nutr* 1993; 57:146-53; The National Diet-Heart Study Final Report. *Circulation* 1968; 37:I1-428; Sheppard L, Kristal AR, Kushi LH. Weight loss in women participating in a randomized trial of low-fat diets. *Am J Clin Nutr* 1991; 54:821-8.

32.   *In the late 1970s, just about the time the low-fat craze...* Stephen AM, Wald NJ. Trends in individual consumption of dietary fat in the United States, 1920-1984. *Am J of Clin Nutr* 1990; 52:457-69.

32.   *By the mid-1990s, that figure was down to 34* percent. Daily Dietary Fat and Total Food-Energy Intakes—Third National Health and Nutrition Examination Survey, Phase 1, 1988-91. *MMWR* 1994; 43:116-17.

32.   *Yet over the same time, the percentage of obese Americans soared...* Kuczmarski RJ, Flegal KM, Campbell SM, Johnson CL. Increasing prevalence of overweight among US adults. The National Health and Nutrition Examination Surveys, 1960 to 1991 [see comments]. *JAMA* 1994; 272:205-11.

32.   *After the medical definition of obesity changed in 1998...* National Center for Health Statistics, June 1998.

32.   *In 1990 the U.S. government "challenged" food manufacturers...* U.S.HHS, *Healthy People 2000.* Washington, DC: U.S. Government Printing Office, 1990

32.   *The National Cholesterol Education Program is still encouraging...* National Cholesterol Education Program. Second Report of the Expert Panel on Detection, Evaluation, and Treatment of High Blood Cholesterol in Adults (Adult Treatment Panel II). *Circulation* 1994; 89:1333-445.

32.   *...and the American Heart Association says...* American Heart Association web page: www.americanheart.org, under "Fat Substitutes."

33.   *Since the 1970s Americans have added an extra twenty-eight pounds of sugar...*Putman JJ, Allshouse JE. *Food consumption, prices and expenditure, 1970-95.* Washington, DC: USDA, 1997.

33. *Nielsen ratings reveal they spend at least...* Historical Daily Viewing Activity. Nielson Media Research, 1998. 299 Park Ave, NY, NY

33. *With the exception of the American Diabetes Association...* Franz MJ, Horton ES, Sr., Bantle JP, et al. Nutrition principles for the management of diabetes and related complications. *Diabetes Care* 1994; 17:490-518.

Chapter 3: Diets That Do Work

35. *An NIH Panel estimated their failure....* Methods for voluntary weight loss and control. NIH Technology Assessment Conference Panel. *Annals of Internal Medicine* 1993; 119:764-770.

36. *Today, according to anthropologist Sidney Mintz...* Keiger D. Matters of Taste. *Johns Hopkins Magazine* 1998; November:12-18.

Chapter 4: Cancer, Fat, and Low-Fat Diets

41. *In the National Cancer Institute's...* Action Guide for Healthy Eating. NCI, NIH Publication No. 95-3877, 1995.

43. *Some diets, including some low-fat diets, can promote oxidation...* Adam O, Lemmen C, Kless T, Adam P, Denzlinger C, Hailer S. Low fat diet decreases alpha-tocopherol levels, and stimulates LDL oxidation and eicosanoid biosynthesis in man. *Eur J Med Res* 1995; 1:65-71; Sarkkinen ES, Uusitupa MI, Nyyssonen K, Parviainen M, Penttila I, Salonen JT. Effects of two low-fat diets, high and low in polyunsaturated fatty acids, on plasma lipid peroxides and serum vitamin E levels in free-living hypercholesterolaemic men. *Eur J Clin Nutr* 1993; 47:623-30.

46. *When we surveyed a group of physicians...* Vigilante K, Flynn, M, unpublished data.

47. *Experiments in animals suggest that polyunsaturated fats...* Rose DP. Dietary fatty acids and cancer. *Am J Clin Nutr* 1997; 66:998S-1003S.

47. *It is the ultimate nutritional irony that these fats...* National Cholesterol Education Program. Second Report of the Expert Panel on Detection, Evaluation, and Treatment of High Blood Cholesterol in Adults (Adult Treatment Panel II). *Circulation* 1994; 89:1333-445.

49. *Famous for their role in preventing heart disease, omega-3 fatty acids...* Rose DP. Dietary fatty acids and cancer. *Am J Clin Nutr* 1997; 66:998S-1003S.

49. *While not strongly associated with cancer...* Kohlmeier L, Simonsen N, van 't Veer P, et al. Adipose tissue trans fatty acids and breast can-

cer in the European Community Multicenter Study on Antioxidants, Myocardial Infarction, and Breast Cancer [see comments]. *Cancer Epidemiol Biomarkers Prev* 1997; 6:705-10.

53. *But the biggest health problem with olestra....* Stampfer M. Effects of carotenoid reduction on disease incidence: quantitative estimates. In: Anderson D, ed. *Potential effects of reducing carotenoid levels on human health.* Harvard School of Public Health; 1996:71-76.

53. *Dr. Meir Stampfer of the Harvard School...* Stampfer M. Effects of carotenoid reduction on disease incidence: quantitative estimates. In: Anderson D, ed. *Potential effects of reducing carotenoid levels on human health.* Harvard School of Public Health; 1996:71-76.

54. *Carotenoids can be divided into carotenes or oxycarotenoids.* Krinsky NI. Carotenoids: Structure and functions, *Proceedings of the Workshop. Potential effects of reducing carotenoid levels on human health,* Harvard School of Public Health, January 17, 1996.

54. *At least one study has shown that carotenes may help...* Krinsky NI. Carotenoids: Structure and functions, *Proceedings of the Workshop. Potential effects of reducing carotenoid levels on human health,* Harvard School of Public Health, January 17, 1996.

54. *Other research suggests carotenes encourage cells...* Amir H, al e. Lycopene synergizes with 1,25 (OH)2 vitamin-D3 in the inhibition of cell cycle progression and the induction of differentiation in leukemia cell (abstract*), Eleventh International Symposium on Carotenoids, The Netherlands,* 1996; Levy J, al. e. Lycopene inhibits cancer cell proliferation by delaying cell cycle progression in G1 phases (abstract), *Eleventh International Symposium on Carotenoids, The Netherlands,* 1996.

55. *But carotenes have another property that distinguishes...* Williams AW, Boileau TW, Erdman JW, Jr. Factors influencing the uptake and absorption of carotenoids. *Proc Soc Exp Biol Med* 1998; 218:106-8.

56. *A number of studies have shown that vitamin E....* Diaz MN, Frei B, Vita JA, Keaney JF, Jr. Antioxidants and atherosclerotic heart disease. *N Engl J Med* 1997;337:408-16; Knekt P, Aromaa A, Maatela J, et al. Vitamin E and cancer prevention. *Am J Clin Nutr* 1991 53:283S-286S.

57. *The authors of an NCI document... Cancer Rates and Risks.* Harras A, ed. Washington, DC: U.S. Department f Health and Human Services, 1996:205.

57. *In fact, in the U.S. where olive oil is not that widely consumed...* Block G, Dresser CM, Hartman AM, Carroll MD. Nutrient sources in the American diet: Quantitative data from the NHANES II Study. *Am J of Epidemiol* 1985; 122:27-40.

58. *And when meat or fish is cooked so that it is seared...* Weisburger JH. Dietary fat and risk of chronic disease: mechanistic insights from experimental studies. *J Am Diet Assoc* 1997; 97:S16-S23.

59. *However, it has recently been discovered that olive oil contains...* Steinmetz KA, Potter JD. Vegetables, fruits, and cancer. II. Mechanisms. *Cancer Causes and Control* 1991; 2:427-442.

59. *Olive oil has still other phytochemicals...*Oguri A, Suda M, Totsuka Y, Sugimura T, Wakabayashi K. Inhibitory effects of antioxidants on formation of heterocyclic amines. *Mutat Res* 1998; 402:237-45.

60. *Although in population studies fat intake of all kinds...*Weisburger JH. Dietary fat and risk of chronic disease: mechanistic insights from experimental studies. *J Am Diet Assoc* 1997; 97:S16-S23.

60. *A recent study showed that eating well-done meat...* Aheng We, Gustafson DR, Sinha R, et al. Well-done meat intake and the risk of breast cancer. *J Natl Cancer Institute* 1998; 90:1724-1729.

60. *In very large studies of women living in the United States and Europe...*Willett WC. Diet and health: what should we eat? *Science* 1994; 264:532-7.

60. *In Greece, Italy, and Spain, where the consumption of fat...*Willet W. *Overview of Nutritional Epidemiology.* Nutrition Epidemiology. Vol. 30, Chapter 16, Dietary Fat and Breast Cancer. New York: Oxford University Press, 1998.

61. *One of the best-kept secrets about carotenes...* Handelman G. Physiological effects of carotenoids in humans. In: Anderson D, ed. *Potential effects of reducing carotenoid levels on human health,* Harvard School of Public Health; 1996:18-23.

62. *On the other hand, in five recent studies...*Willett W, Hunter D, Stampfer M, al e. Dietary fat and fiber in relation to risk of breast cancer: an 8 year follow-up. *JAMA* 1992; 268:2037-2044; Landa MC, Frago N, Tres A. Diet and the risk of breast cancer in Spain. *Eur J Cancer Prev* 1994; 3:313-20; Martin-Moreno JM, Willett WC, Gorgojo L, et al. Dietary fat, olive oil intake and breast cancer risk. *Int J Cancer* 1994; 58:774-80; Trichopolous A, Katsouyanni K, Stuver S, et al. Consumption of olive oil and specific food groups in relation to breast cancer risk in Greece [see comments]. *J Natl Cancer Inst* 1995; 87:110-6; la Vecchia C, Negri E, Franceschi S, Decarli A, Giacosa A, Lipworth L. Olive oil, other dietary fats, and the risk of breast cancer (Italy). *Cancer Causes Control* 1995; 6:545-50; Wolk A, Bergstrom R, Hunter D, et al. A prospective study of association of monounsaturated fat and other types of fat with risk of breast cancer [see comments]. *Arch Intern Med* 1998; 158:41-5.

62. *The evidence shows that breast cancer is more likely...* Greenwald P, Sherwood K, McDonald SS. Fat, caloric intake, and obesity: lifestyle risk factors for breast cancer. *J Am Diet Assoc* 1997; 97:S24-30.

62. *Dr. Walter Willett exhaustively reviewed the issue...*Willet W. *Overview of Nutritional Epidemiology.* Vol. 30. New York: Oxford University Press, 1998. Quote on page 406.

63. *It has been shown that men who eat more marinara...* Giovannucci E, Clinton SK. Tomatoes, lycopene, and prostate cancer. *Proc Soc Exp Biol Med* 1998; 218:129-39.

63. *And as Dr. Antonia Trichopoulou of the University of Athens...*Mediterranean Diet Conference, January 1998. Oldways Preservation & Exchange Trust. 25 First Street, Cambridge, MA 02141.

63. *Otherwise it would be very hard to explain why heavy smoking...* Keys A. Coronary heart disease in seven countries. *Circulation* 1970; 41:1-211; *Food, Nutrition and the Prevention of Cancer: a global perspective,* World Cancer Research Fund in Association with American Institute for Cancer Research, 1997.

Chapter 5: Can Low-Fat Diets Worsen Your Cholesterol?

66. *The low-fat diet has been the cornerstone...* Dietary goals for the United States: statement of The American Medical Association to the Select Committee on Nutrition and Human Needs, United States Senate. *R I Med J* 1977; 60:576-81.

66. *...but a low-fat diet can also lower your levels of HDL...* Katan MB, Grundy SM, Willett WC. Should a low-fat, high-carbohydrate diet be recommended for everyone? Beyond low-fat diets. *N Engl J Med* 1997; 337:563-6

68. *Actually the cholesterol you eat has very little to do...* McNamara D. Cholesterol intake and plasma cholesterol: an update. *Journal of the American College of Nutrition* 1997; 16:530-534.

68. *Starting in the 1970s, Americans were instructed...* AHA. Diet and Heart Disease. Dallas: American Heart Association, 1973.

69. *Another recent theory is that HDL promotes other substances...*Vinals M, Martinez-Gonzalez J, Badimon L. Mechanism of Prostacyclin Upregulation by HDL. *Circulation* 1998; 98:2830.

69. *Unfortunately, the dietary advice most doctors gave to lower LDL...* Katan MB, Grundy SM, Willett WC. Should a low-fat, high-carbohydrate diet be recommended for everyone? Beyond low-fat diets [see comments]. *N Engl J Med* 1997; 337:563-6; Katan MB. Effect of low-fat diets on plasma high-density lipoprotein concentrations. *Am J Clin Nutr* 1998; 67:573S-576S.

70. *Eighty-two percent of the physicians....* Vigilante K, Flynn M. Inadequate physician knowledge of the effect of diet on blood lipids. *Circulation* 1998; 98:3075.

70. *Recent research suggests that in some people...* Krauss RM, Dreon DM. Low- density-lipoprotein subclasses and response to a low-fat diet in healthy men. *Am J Clin Nutr* 1995; 62:478S-487S.

71. *It is these small oxidized LDL particles...* O'Keefe JH, Jr., Lavie CJ, Jr., McCallister BD. Insights into the pathogenesis and prevention of coronary artery disease. *Mayo Clin Proc* 1995; 70:69-79.

73. *In a recent experiment Dr. Ron Krauss...* Krauss RM, Dreon DM. Low-density-lipoprotein subclasses and response to a low-fat diet in healthy men. *Am J Clin Nutr* 1995; 62:478S-487S.

74. *When we asked what size cholesterol....*Vigilante K, Flynn M. Inadequate physician knowledge of the effect of diet on blood lipids. *Circulation* 1998; 98:3075.

74. *The 25 percent fat mark appears to be a critical lower boundary...* Brussard J, Katan M, Groot P, Havekes L, JGAJ H. Serum lipoproteins of healthy persons fed a low-fat diet or a polyunsaturated fat diet for three months. *Atherosclerosis* 1982; 42:205-219; Knopp RH, Walden CE, Retzlaff BM, et al. Long-term cholesterol-lowering effects of 4 fat-restricted diets in hypercholesterolemic and combined hyperlipidemic men. The Dietary Alternatives Study [see comments]. *JAMA* 1997; 278:1509-15.

75. *Only in the summer of 1998 did the American Heart...* Lichtenstein AH, Van Horn L. Very low fat diets. *Circulation* 1998; 98:935-9.

75. *Sixty percent felt that a "low-fat diet"...*Vigilante K, Flynn M. Inadequate physician knowledge of the effect of diet on blood lipids. *Circulation* 1998; 98:3075.

75. *Some low-fat proponents like Dean Ornish...*Ornish D. *Eat more, weigh less.* First ed. New York: HarperPerennial; 1994:424.

75. *Very-low-fat diets may impair your absorption....*Handelman G. Physiological effects of carotenoids in humans. In: Anderson D, ed. *Potential effects of reducing carotenoid levels on human health.* Harvard School of Public Health; 1996:18-23.

Chapter 6: The Danger Your Doctor Doesn't Talk About

77. *In fact, as recently as 1996 the American College of Physicians...* Guidelines for using serum cholesterol, high-density lipoprotein cholesterol, and triglyceride levels as screening tests for preventing coronary heart disease in adults. *Annals of Internal Medicine* 1996; 124:515-517.

78. *The government-sponsored National Cholesterol Education Program says...* National Cholesterol Education Program. Second Report of the Expert Panel on Detection, Evaluation, and Treatment of High Blood Cholesterol in Adults (Adult Treatment Panel II). *Circulation* 1994; 89:1333-445.

78. *For instance, Dr. Jorgen Jeppesen and his colleagues...* Jeppesen J, Hein HO, Suadicani P, Gyntelberg F. Triglyceride concentration and ischemic heart disease: an eight-year follow-up in the Copenhagen Male Study. *Circulation* 1998; 97:1029-36.

78. *In another recent study of heart patients...* Miller M. Is hypertriglyceridaemia an independent risk factor for coronary heart disease? The epidemiological evidence. *Eur Heart J* 1998; 19 Suppl H:H18-22.

79. *Well, when you have a high fasting level of triglycerides...* Grundy SM. Small LDL, atherogenic dyslipidemia, and the metabolic syndrome. *Circulation* 1997; 95:1-4; McNamara JR, Jenner JL, Li Z, Wilson PW, Schaefer EJ. Change in LDL particle size is associated with change in plasma triglyceride concentration. *Arterioscler Thromb* 1992; 12:1284-90.

80. *LDL that is extra rich in triglyceride attracts...* Zambon A, Austin MA, Brown BG, Hokanson JE, Brunzell JD. Effect of hepatic lipase on LDL in normal men and those with coronary artery disease. *Arterioscler Thromb* 1993; 13:147-53.

80. *In 1992 Dr. William Castelli,...* Castelli WP. Epidemiology of triglycerides: a view from Framingham. *Am J Cardiol* 1992; 70:3H-9H.

81. *It's a low-fat, high-carb diet, especially if you do not lose weight...* Mensink RP, Katan MB. Effect of monounsaturated fatty acids versus complex carbohydrates on high-density lipoproteins in healthy men and women. *Lancet* 1987; 1:122-5; Grundy SM. Comparison of monounsaturated fatty acids and carbohydrates for lowering plasma cholesterol. *N Engl J Med* 1986; 314:745-8.

81. *We conducted a survey of physicians...* Vigilante K, Flynn M. Inadequate physician knowledge of the effect of diet on blood lipids. *Circulation* 1998; 98.

81. *How does a high-carb diet raise triglycerides?* Farquhar JW, Frank A, Gross RC, Reaven GM. Glucose, insulin, and triglyceride responses to high and low carbohydrate diets in man. *J Clin Invest* 1966; 45:1648-56.

81. *When we asked doctors what would happen to someone...* Vigilante K, Flynn M., unpublished survey results.

82. *This claim is based on exactly one study...* Antonis A, Bersohn I. The

influence of diet on serum-triglycerides in South African white and Bantu prisoners. *Lancet* 1961:3-9.

82. *A recent study by coauthor Dr. Mary Flynn...* Flynn MM, Zmuda JM, Milosavljevic D, Caldwell MJ, Herbert PN. Lipoprotein response to a National Cholesterol Education Program Step II Diet with and without energy restriction. *Metabolism* 1999; (in press).

84. *By replacing some carbohydrate calories with olive oil...* Baggio G, Pagnan A, Muraca M, et al. Olive-oil-enriched diet: effect on serum lipoprotein levels and biliary cholesterol saturation. *Am J Clin Nutr* 1988; 47:960-4; Berry EM, Eisenberg S, Friedlander Y, et al. Effects of diets rich in monounsaturated fatty acids on plasma lipoproteins—the Jerusalem Nutrition Study. II. Monounsaturated fatty acids vs carbohydrates. *Am J Clin Nutr* 1992; 56:394-403.

Chapter 7: Low-Fat Diets and the Silent Killer

88. *People who carry their fat around their waist...* Sjostrom LV. Mortality of severely obese people. *Am J Clin Nutr* 1992; 55:516S-523S.

88. *With more than 50 percent of the American population...* Kuczmarski RJ, Carroll MD, Flegal KM, Troiano RP. Varying body mass index cutoff points to describe overweight prevalence among U.S. adults: NHANES III (1988 to 1994). *Obes Res* 1997; 5:542-8.

88. *The good news is that losing just 5 to 10 percent...* Goldstein DJ. Beneficial health effects of modest weight loss. *Int J Obes Relat Metab Disord* 1992; 16:397-415.

89. *Approximately two-thirds of the physicians...*Vigilante K, Flynn M. Inadequate physician knowledge of the effect of diet on blood lipids. *Circulation* 1998; 98.

90. *Worse, our research showed...*Vigilante K, Flynn M. Inadequate physician knowledge of the effect of diet on blood lipids. *Circulation.* 1998;98:3075.

90. *Scientists from Spain found that HDL...*Vinals M, Martinez-Gonzalez J, Badimon L. Mechanism of prostacyclin upregulation by HDL. *Circulation* 1998; 98:(abs) 2830.

93. *Between 1987 and 1994, death from heart disease went down...*Rosamond WD, Chambless LE, Folsom AR, et al. Trends in the incidence of myocardial infarction and in mortality due to coronary heart disease, 1987 to 1994. *N Engl J Med* 1998; 339:861-7.

94. *As Scott Grundy has said, "there is a growing realization...* Grundy SM. Multifactorial causation of obesity: implications for prevention. *Am J Clin Nutr* 1998; 67:563S-72S.

Chapter 8: Dean Ornish: King of the Fat Phobes

95. *Ornish doesn't want a drop of olive oil to touch ...* Ornish D. *Eat more, weigh less.* First ed. New York: HarperPerennial; 1994. P. 35.

96. *In 1990 Dr. Ornish and his colleagues published...* Ornish D, Brown SE, Scherwitz LW, et al. Can lifestyle changes reverse coronary heart disease? The Lifestyle Heart Trial. *Lancet* 1990; 336:129-33.

97. *But as food critic Jeffrey Steingarten....* Steingarten J. *The Man Who Ate Everything.* New York: Alfred A. Knopf; 1997.

97. *He asserts that his no-fat diet "is the most effective diet for lowering"...* Ornish D. Dr. Dean Ornish's program for reversing heart disease: the only system scientifically proven to reverse heart disease without drugs or surgery. 1st ed. New York: Random House; 1990:xx, 631.

99. *To put it in perspective only about 4 percent...* Crespo CJ, Keteyian SJ, Heath GW, Sempos CT. Leisure-time physical activity among US adults. Results from the Third National Health and Nutrition Examination Survey. *Arch Intern Med* 1996; 156:93-8.

99. *For instance, doctors from Heidelberg, Germany...* Hambrecht R, Niebauer J, Marburger C, et al. Various intensities of leisure time physical activity in patients with coronary artery disease: effects on cardiorespiratory fitness and progression of coronary atherosclerotic lesions. *J Am Coll Cardiol* 1993; 22:468-77; Niebauer J, Hambrecht R, Velich T, et al. Attenuated progression of coronary artery disease after 6 years of multifactorial risk intervention: role of physical exercise. *Circulation* 1997; 96:2534-41.

99. *Exercise tends to raise HDL...* Thompson PD, Yurgalevitch SM, Flynn MM, et al. Effect of prolonged exercise training without weight loss on high-density lipoprotein metabolism in overweight men. *Metabolism* 1997; 46:217-23.

100. *Weight loss alone seems to have independent beneficial effects...* Dattilo AM, Kris-Etherton PM. Effects of weight reduction on blood lipids and lipoproteins: a meta-analysis. A J Clin Nut 1992; 56:320-8; Goldstein DJ. Beneficial health effects of modest weight loss. *Int J Obes Relat Metab Disord* 1992; 16:397-415.

100. *Reducing stress and negative emotions...* Cooper MJ, Aygen MM. A relaxation technique in the management of hypercholesterolemia. *J Human Stress* 1979; 5:24-7; Patel C, Marmot MG, Terry DJ, Carruthers M, Hunt B, Patel M. Trial of relaxation in reducing coronary risk: four year follow up. *Br Med J* (Clin Res Ed) 1985; 290:1103-6.

101. *Some of his patients became so fat phobic...* Personal communication with Preventive Medicine Research Institute. December 17, 1998.

103. *Ornish ignores the healthy Mediterranean diet data...* Ornish D. *Eat more, weigh less.* New York: HarperPerennial, 1994:424.

103. *Unfortunately, that excludes about 95 percent of U.S. adults...* Brown S, Hutchinson R, Morrisett J, et al. Plasma lipid, lipoprotein cholesterol, and apoprotein distributions in selected US communities. The Atherosclerosis Risk in Communities (ARIC) Study. *Arterioscler and Thromb* 1993;13:1139-1158.

103. *In his book* Everyday cooking with Dr. Dean Ornish *he gets specific with his attack on olive...* Ornish D. *Everyday cooking with Dr. Dean Ornish.* New York: HarperCollins, 1997: 5.

103. *Unfortunately, Dr. Ornish doesn't know the scientific evidence...* Grundy SM. Comparison of monounsaturated fatty acids and carbohydrates for lowering plasma cholesterol. *N Engl J Med* 1986; 314:745-8; Mensink RP, Katan MB. Effect of monounsaturated fatty acids versus complex carbohydrates on high-density lipoproteins in healthy men and women. *Lancet* 1987; 1:122-5.

104. *...citing studies showing that these diets....* Danforth E, Jr., Horton ES, O'Connell M, et al. Dietary-induced alterations in thyroid hormone metabolism during overnutrition *J Clin Invest* 1979; 64:1336-47; Mathieson RA, Walberg JL, Gwazdauskas FC, Hinkle DE, Gregg JM. The effect of varying carbohydrate content of a very-low-caloric diet on resting metabolic rate and thyroid hormones. *Metabolism* 1986; 35:394-8; Spaulding SW, Chopra IJ, Sherwin RS, Lyall SS. Effect of caloric restriction and dietary composition of serum T3 and reverse T3 in man. *J Clin Endocrinol Metab* 1976; 42:197- 200.

104. *But in the one study that actually measured metabolic rate...* Mathieson RA, Walberg JL, Gwazdauskas FC, Hinkle DE, Gregg JM. The effect of varying carbohydrate content of a very-low-caloric diet on resting metabolic rate and thyroid hormones. *Metabolism* 1986; 35:394-8.

104. *Insulin goes down when you lose weight.* Riccardi G, Parillo M. Comparison of the metabolic effects of fat-modified vs low fat diets. *Ann N Y Acad Sci* 1993; 683:192-8.

104. *Again in reality, the study shows something different than what -...*Chen J, Campbell T, Tunyao L, Peto R. *Diet, lifestyle and mortality in China: a study of the characteristics of 65 chinese countries.* Oxford: Oxford University Press, 1990. Tables 5005 and 5008

105. *Studies have shown that even highly motivated people have a hard time...* Knopp RH, Walden CE, Retzlaff BM, et al. Long-term cholesterol-

lowering effects of 4 fat-restricted diets in hypercholesterolemic and combined hyperlipidemic men. The Dietary Alternatives Study. *JAMA*. 1997;278:1509-15.

106. *Had Ornish done this, as Dr. Frank Sachs,...*Sacks FM, Willett, WC. Lipid Levels and "Affluent Diets". *N Engl J Med* 1992; 327:54 (letter).

106. *Results of the Nurses' Health Study reveal that women..* Hu F, Stampfer M, Manson J, et al. Frequent nut consumption and risk of coronary heart disease: prospective cohort study. *British Medical Journal.* 1998;317:1341-1345.

106. *The Lyon heart study in France showed a dramatic reduction...*Renaud S, de Lorgeril M, Delaye J, et al. Cretan Mediterranean diet for prevention of coronary heart disease. *Am J Clin Nutr* 1995; 61:1360S-1367S.

106. *And even more impressive, five years later...*de Lorgeril M, Salen P, Martin JL, Monjaud I, Boucher P, Mamelle N. Mediterranean dietary pattern in a randomized trial: prolonged survival and possible reduced cancer rate. *Arch Intern Med.* 1998; 158:1181-7.

107. *This is the experience of a reporter, Gina Kolata, who went to dinner with Dr. Ornish.* New York Times, December 29, 1998.

Chapter 9: The High-Fat Fraud

111. *When insulin is high, LPL at the muscle...* Eckel RH. Lipoprotein lipase. A multifunctional enzyme relevant to common metabolic diseases. *N Engl J Med* 1989; 320:1060-8.

114. *This study purported to show that among a group of patients...* Kekwick A, Pawan GLS. Calorie intake in relation to body-weight changes in the obese. *Lancet* 1956:155-161.

115. *Those extra purloined calories could easily account...* A critique of low-carbohydrate ketogenic weight reduction regimens. *JAMA* 1973; 224:1415-1419.

115. *The glycemic index, a scale developed by Jenkins...* Jenkins DJ, Wolever TM, Taylor RH, et al. Glycemic index of foods: a physiological basis for carbohydrate exchange. *Am J Clin Nutr* 1981; 34:362-6.

115. *So powerful is the all mighty Zone that...* Sears B, Ph.D. *The zone: a revolutionary life plan to put your body in total balance for permanent weight loss.* New York: Regan Books, 1995:286 (book cover).

116. *As previously mentioned, elevated insulin...* Sjostrom LV. Morbidity of severely obese subjects. *Am J Clin Nutr* 1992; 55:508S-515S.

116. *Sears's error is probably why Dr. Gerald Reaven...*Gladwell M. The Pima Paradox. *The New Yorker* 1998:44-57.

116. *However, they fail to adequately emphasize that these foods are rarely eaten in isolation...* Bornet FR, Costagliola D, Rizkalla SW, et al. Insulinemic and glycemic indexes of six starch-rich foods taken alone and in a mixed meal by type 2 diabetics. *Am J Clin Nutr* 1987; 45:588-95.

117. *Researchers at Duke University put one group...* Surwit RS, Feinglos MN, McCaskill CC, et al. Metabolic and behavioral effects of a high-sucrose diet during weight loss. *Am J Clin Nutr* 1997; 65:908-15.

118. *In our survey, 65 percent..* Vigilante K, Flynn M. Inadequate physician knowledge of the effect of diet on blood lipids. *Circulation.* 1998; 98:3075.

118. *Kerns did exactly what Barry Sears...* Kerns MA. Effects of two energy restriction diets on fuel utilization, blood chemistry and body composition. *Medicine and Science in Sports and Exercise* 1998; 30:s62 (abstract).

120. *Dr. Agaston, a cardiologist at the Mt. Sinai Medical Center...* Lopez-Jimenez F, Heilbron R, Altman M, Korn H, Lamas GA, Agatston AS. The beneficial effect of a high-fat, high-protein, low-carbohydrate diet on body weight and HDL cholesterol. *J Am Coll Card* 1998; 31:88A.

122. *Weight loss causes blood cholesterol to drop...* Dattilo AM, Kris-Etherton PM. Effects of weight reduction on blood lipids and lipoproteins: a meta-analysis. *Am J Clin Nutr* 1992; 56:320-8.

122. *First, protein leaches calcium...* Nordin BE. International patterns of osteoporosis. *Clin Orthop* 1966; 45:17-30; Lutz J, Linkswiler HM. Calcium metabolism in postmenopausal and osteoporotic women consuming two levels of dietary protein. *Am J Clin Nutr* 1981; 34:2178-86.

122. *Second, excess meat consumption, the biggest source of protein, is associated with heart disease...* Phillips RL, Lemon FR, Beeson WL, Kuzma JW. Coronary heart disease mortality among Seventh-Day Adventists with differing dietary habits: a preliminary report. *Am J Clin Nutr* 1978; 31:S191-S198.

122. *...excess meat consumption... is associated with... and cancer...* Willett WC, Stampfer MJ, Colditz GA, Rosner BA, Speizer FE. Relation of meat, fat, and fiber intake to the risk of colon cancer in a prospective study among women. *N Engl J Med* 1990; 323:1664-72; Le Marchand L, Kolonel LN, Wilkens LR, Myers BC, Hirohata T. Animal fat consumption and prostate cancer: a prospective study in Hawaii. *Epidemiology* 1994; 5:276-82.

122. *...and recent evidence has convincingly linked well-cooked meat to breast cancer...* Zheng W, Gustafson DR, Sinha R, et al. Well-done meat intake and the risk of breast cancer. J N Can Inst 1998; 90:1724-17229.

122. *Finally, there is even some evidence that protein can bind...* Hertog M, Katan M. Quercetin in foods, cardiovascular disease, and cancer. In: Rice-Evans CA, Packer L, eds. *Flavonoids in Health and Disease.* New York: Marcel Dekker, Inc., 1998:21.

Chapter 10: Eat Fast Food, Die Younger, Leave an Obese Corpse

125. *Fast food is a $103 billion industry...* Parade, November 16, 1997.

126. *Approximately 30 percent of American children are obese...* Mellin L. To: President Clinton, Re: combating childhood obesity. *J Am Diec Assoc* 1993; 93:265-266.

126. *A study sponsored by the National Research Council....* Branigin, Willian. Fitting in leaves children less fit. American lifestyles take toll on young immigrants' health. *Washington Post,* September 10, 1998, p. A01.

127. *But fast-food chains are now contracting with public schools...* School lunches, fast food in the lunchroom. *Consumer Reports,* September 1998.

127. *According to* Rolling Stone *magazine...* Fast Food Nation, *Rolling Stone,* September 3, 1998, p. 61.

130. *(By the way, virgin olive oil is remarkably...* Luchetti F. Olive Oil and Health. Spain: International Olive Oil Council; 1997.

Chapter 11: Fraud Foods

131. *Like saturated fats trans fats raise LDL...* Blume E. Hydrogenation: The Food Industry's Wild Card. *Nutrition Action* 1987:8-9; Katan MB, Zock PL, Mensink RP. Trans fatty acids and their effects on lipoproteins in humans. *Annu Rev Nutr* 1995; 15:473-93.

132. *In the Nurses Health Study, women who consumed...* Willet W. *Overview of Nutritional Epidemiology.* Diet and Coronary Heart Disease. Vol. 30. Chapter 17. New York: Oxford University Press, 1998.

132. *ConAgra is a multimllion-dollar food manufacturing behemoth.* ConAgra web page: www.conagra.com. January 1999.

133. *Of the physicians responding to our survey, a shocking 69 percent...* Vigilante K, Flynn M, unpublished survey results.

136. *Today, they represent 3 to 5 percent of calories.* Allison DB, Egan SK, Barraj LM, Caughman C, Infante M, Heimbach JT. Estimated intakes of trans fatty and other fatty acids in the US population. *J Am Diet Assoc* 1999; 99:166-74; quiz 175-6. Willett WC. Diet and health: what should we eat? *Science* 1994; 264:532-7.

136. *Dr Martin Katan, the internationally famous lipid researcher...* Plenary Session XI: Lifestyle Choices and New Pharmacologic Approaches to Prevention of Cardiovascular Disease, American Heart Association Meeting, Dallas, Texas. November 1998.

Chapter 12: The Healthiest Diet in the World

141. *But the healthiest diet in the western world...* Nestle M. Mediterranean diets: historical and research overview. *Am J Clin Nutr* 1995; 61:1313S-1320S

141. *In the early 1950s, researcher Leland Albaugh...* Nestle M. Mediterranean diets: historical and research overview. *Am J Clin Nutr* 1995; 61:1313S-1320S.

141. *In the 1961 census data on Greece...*Nestle M. Mediterranean diets: historical and research overview. *Am J Clin Nutr* 1995; 61:1313S-1320S.

142. *At a 1952 nutrition conference in Rome...* Keys A. Mediterranean diet and public health: personal reflections. *Am J Clin Nutr* 1995; 61:1321S-1323S.

142. *The low heart-disease rates in Naples ...* Keys A. Coronary heart disease in seven countries. *Circulation* 1970; 41:1-211.

143. *A report published in 1998 reveals that Spain...* Bosch X. Spanish live long and healthy lives. *Lancet.* 1998; 352:1610.

143. *In 1984 a fifteen-year analysis was published...* Keys A, Menotti A, Aravanis C, et al. The seven countries study: 2,289 deaths in 15 years. *Prev Med* 1984; 13:141-54.

145. *In 1986 another follow-up analysis...* Keys A, Menotti A, Karvonen MJ, et al. The diet and 15-year death rate in the seven countries study. *Am J Epidemiol* 1986; 124:903-15.

145. *For instance, women of Toulouse...* Renaud S, de Lorgeril M, Delaye J, et al. Cretan Mediterranean diet for prevention of coronary heart disease. *Am J Clin Nutr.* 1995; 61:1360S-1367S.

146. *Spaniards as a whole are second....* Bosch X. Spanish live long and healthy lives. *Lancet* 1998; 352:1610.

146. *Dr. Antonia Trichopoulou studied...*Trichopoulou A, Kouris-Blazos A,

Vassilakou T, et al. Diet and survival of elderly Greeks: a link to the past. *Am J Clin Nutr* 1995; 61:1346S-1350S.

146. *Dr. Henry Blackburn, a world-famous expert...* Renaud S, de Lorgeril M, Delaye J, et al. Cretan Mediterranean diet for prevention of coronary heart disease. *Am J Clin Nutr* 1995; 61:1360S-1367S.

147. *The following is Dr. Ancel Keys's observations...* Nestle M. Mediterranean diets: historical and research overview. *Am J Clin Nutr* 1995; 61:1313S-1320S.

147. *Recently a group of French doctors...* Renaud S, de Lorgeril M, Delaye J, et al. Cretan Mediterranean diet for prevention of coronary heart disease. *Am J Clin Nutr* 1995; 61:1360S-1367S.

149. *Renaud continued to follow the original participants...*de Lorgeril M, Salen P, Martin JL, Monjaud I, Boucher P, Mamelle N. Mediterranean dietary pattern in a randomized trial: prolonged survival and possible reduced cancer rate. *Arch Intern Med* 1998; 158:1181-7.

150. *In Keys's study the Japanese were second...* Keys A. Coronary heart disease in seven countries. *Circulation* 1970; 41:1-211.

150. *Only about 6 percent of those studied were considered sedentary...* Keys A. Coronary heart disease in seven countries. *Circulation* 1970; 41:1-211.

151. *We know from studies like the one published in...* Knopp RH, Walden CE, Retzlaff BM, et al. Long-term cholesterol-lowering effects of 4 fat-restricted diets in hypercholesterolemic and combined hyperlipidemic men. The Dietary Alternatives Study. *JAMA* 1997; 278:1509-15.

153. *This is probably because Japan has topped the longevity charts...*World Health Statistics Annual. Geneva: World Health Organization.

154. *According to food reformer Dun Gifford, one of the early skirmishes was fought by...* Personal communication with K. Dun Gifford, Oldways Preservation and Exchange Trust, Cambridge, MA. August 1998.

154. *The Senate Select Committee on Nutrition and Human Needs...* Hearings before the Select Committee on Nutrition and Human Needs of the United States Senate. Ninety-fourth Congress. Second Session 1976 and First Session 1977.U.S. Government Printing Office, Washington.

154. *...and issued a report that contained the first federal dietary recommendations...* Dietary goals for the United States: statement of The American Medical Association to the Select Committee on Nutrition and Human Needs, United States Senate. *R I Med J.* 1977;60:576-81.

154. *Unfortunately it provoked an uproar from the meat industry...* Nestle M. Dietary advice for the 1990s: the political history of the Food Guide Pyramid. *Caduceus* 1993; 9:136-53

155. *Over the years the national data from Japan...*Willett WC. Diet and health: what should we eat? *Science* 1994; 264:532-7.

155. *Japan also has disproportionately high cancer rates....* Willett WC. Diet and health: what should we eat? *Science* 1994; 264:532-7.

Chapter 13: Nature's Healthiest Oil

For general information and materials on olive oil: The Olive Oil Council. Foodcom, Inc., 708 Third Avenue, New York, NY 10017. 212-297-0136

160. *In some cases the speed of oxidation...* Luchetti F. Olive Oil and Health. Spain: International Olive Oil Council, 1997:64.

160. *Caffeic acid:* Aziz NH, Farag SE, Mousa LA, Abo-Zaid MA. Comparative antibacterial and antifungal effects of some phenolic compounds. *Microbios* 1998; 93:43-54; Chan W, Wen P, Chiang H. Structure-activity relationshop of caffeic acid analogues on xanthine oxidase inhibition. *Anticancer Res* 1995; 15:703-707; Galasinski W, Chlabicz J, Paszkiewics-Gadek A, Marcinkiewicz C, Gindzienski A. The substances of plant origin that inhibit protein biosynthesis. *Acta Pol Pharm* 1996; 53:311-318; Laranjinha J, Vieira O, Madeira V, Almeida L. Two related phenolic antioxidants with opposite effects on vitamin E content in low density lipoproteins oxidized by ferrylmyoglobin: consumption vs regeneration. *Arch Biochem Biophys* 1995; 323:373-81; Oguri A, Suda M, Totsuka Y, Sugimura T, Wakabayashi K. Inhibitory effects of antioxidants on formation of heterocyclic amines. *Mutat Res* 1998; 402:237-45; Vieira O, Escargueil-Blanc I, Meilhac O, et al. Effect of dietary phenolic compounds on apoptosis of human cultured endothelial cells induced by oxidized LDL. *Br J Pharmacol* 1998; 123:565-73.

161. *Ferulic acid:* Carbonneau MA, Leger CL, Monnier L, et al. Supplementation with wine phenolic compounds increases the antioxidant capacity of plasma and vitamin E of low-density lipoprotein without changing the lipoprotein $Cu(2+)$-oxidizability: possible explanation by phenolic location. *Eur J Clin Nutr* 1997; 51:682-90; Castelluccio C, Bolwell GP, Gerrish C, Rice-Evans C. Differential distribution of ferulic acid to the major plasma constituents in relation to its potential as an antioxidant. *Biochem J* 1996; 316:691-4. Yamada J, Tomita Y. Antimutagenic activity of caffeic acid and related compounds. *Biosci Biotechnol Biochem* 1996; 60:328-329.

161. *Hydroxytyrosol:* Kohyama N, Nagata T, Fujimoto S, Sekiya K. Inhibition of arachidonate lipoxygenase activities by 2-(3,4- dihydroxyphenyl)ethanol, a phenolic compound from olives. *Biosci Biotechnol Biochem* 1997; 61:347-50; Manna C, Galletti P, Cucciolla V, Moltedo O, Leone A, Zappia V. The protective effect of the olive oil polyphenol (3,4-dihydroxyphenyl)-ethanol counteracts reactive oxygen metabolite-induced cytotoxicity in Caco-2 cells. *J Nutr* 1997; 127:286-92; Petroni A, Blasevich M, Salami M, Papini N, Montedoro GF, Galli C. Inhibition of platelet aggregation and eicosanoid production by phenolic components of olive oil. *Thromb Res* 1995; 78:151-60; Wiseman SA, Mathot JN, de Fouw NJ, Tijburg LB. Dietary non-tocopherol antioxidants present in extra virgin olive oil increase the resistance of low density lipoproteins to oxidation in rabbits. *Atheroscler* 1996; 120:15-23.

161. *Oleuropein:* Aziz NH, Farag SE, Mousa LA, Abo-Zaid MA. Comparative antibacterial and antifungal effects of some phenolic compounds. *Microbios* 1998; 93:43-54.Visioli F, Galli C. Oleuropein protects low density lipoprotein from oxidation. *Life Sci* 1994; 55:1965-71; Visioli F, Bellomo G, Galli C. Free radical-scavenging properties of olive oil polyphenols. *Biochem Biophys Res Commun* 1998; 247:60-4; Visioli F, Bellosta S, Galli C. Oleuropein, the bitter principle of olives, enhances nitric oxide production by mouse macrophages. *Life Sci* 1998; 62:541-6.

161. *Squalene:* Budiarso IT. Fish oil versus olive oil [letter; comment]. *Lancet* 1990; 336:1313-4; Grimes DS, Hindle E, Dyer T. Sunlight, cholesterol and coronary heart disease [see comments]. *Qjm* 1996; 89:579-89; Newmark HL. Squalene, olive oil, and cancer risk: a review and hypothesis. *Cancer Epidemiol Biomarkers Prev* 1997; 6:1101-3

162. *Vanillic acid:* Aziz NH, Farag SE, Mousa LA, Abo-Zaid MA. Comparative antibacterial and antifungal effects of some phenolic compounds. *Microbios* 1998; 93:43-54.

162. *Vitamin E:* Luchetti F. *Olive Oil and Health.* Spain: International Olive Oil Council, 1997:64; Diaz MN, Frei B, Vita JA, Keaney JF, Jr. Antioxidants and atherosclerotic heart disease. *N Engl J Med* 1997; 337:408-16.

163. *Osteoporosis:* Trichopoulou A, Georgiou E, Bassiakos Y, et al. Energy intake and monounsaturated fat in relation to bone mineral density among women and men in Greece. *Prev Med* 1997; 26:395-400.

163. *Cataracts:* Tavani A, Negri E, La Vecchia C. Food and nutrient intake and risk of cataract. *Ann Epidemiol* 1996; 6:41-6.

163. *Arthritis:* Linos A, Kaklamanis E, Kontomerkos A, et al. The effect of olive oil and fish consumption on rheumatoid arthritis—a case control study. *Scand J Rheumatol* 1991; 20:419-26.

163. *Gallbladder disease:* Jonnalagadda S, Trautwein E, Hayes K. Dietary fats rich in saturated fatty aicds (12:0, 14:0, and 16:0) enhance gallstone formation relative to monounsaturated fat (18:1) in cholesterol-fed hamsters. *Lipids* 1995; 30:415-424; Luchetti F. *Olive Oil and Health.* Spain: International Olive Oil Council, 1997:64.

164. *In 1965, when Mademoiselle Jeanne Calmet....* The Economist, August 16, 1997, p. 69.

164. *Hypertension:* Luchetti F. *Olive Oil and Health.* Spain: International Olive Oil Council, 1997:64.

164. *Stroke:* Gillman MW, Cupples LA, Millen BE, Ellison RC. Inverse association of dietary fat with development of ischemic stroke in men. *JAMA* 1997; 278:2145-2150.

167. *In an unfortunate chapter of American history....* New York Times, August 11, 1997, p. A10.

Chapter 14: The Truth about Wine

171. *Despite contradictory evidence in a number of laboratory experiments...* Ridker PM, Vaughan DE, Stampfer MJ, Glynn RJ, Hennekens CH. Association of moderate alcohol consumption and plasma concentration of endogenous tissue-type plasminogen activator. *JAMA* 1994; 272:929-33.

173. *In fact the women in Toulouse...* Renaud S, de Lorgeril M, Delaye J, et al. Cretan Mediterranean diet for prevention of coronary heart disease. *Am J Clin Nutr* 1995; 61:1360S-1367S.

174. *The Copenhagen Heart Study followed...* Gronbaek M, Deis A, Sorensen TI, Becker U, Schnohr P, Jensen G. Mortality associated with moderate intakes of wine, beer, or spirits. *BMJ* 1995; 310:1165-9.

172. *An American Cancer Society survey...* Ellison RC. Here's to your health. Is it now "medically correct" for a physician to prescribe a little wine to lower the risk of heart disease? *Wine Spectator* 1998:35-46.

175. *But some experts maintain that this can account only for...* Rimm EB, Ellison RC. Alcohol in the Mediterranean diet. *Am J Clin Nutr* 1995; 61:1378S-1382S.

175. *Recent evidence suggests that alcohol can also affect the proteins...* Ethanol

stimulates apo A-1 secretion in human hepatocytes: a possible mechanism underlying the cardioprotective effect of ethanol. *Nutr Rev* 1993; 51:151-2.

176. *Other studies suggest that alcohol can inhibit platelets from sticking together...* Pellegrini N, Pareti FI, Stabile F, Brusamolino A, Simonetti P. Effects of moderate consumption of red wine on platelet aggregation and haemostatic variables in healthy volunteers. *Eur J Clin Nutr* 1996; 50:209-13.

176. *A recent study appeared in the* British Medical Journal... Kiechl S, Willeit J, Poewe W, et al. Insulin sensitivity and regular alcohol consumption: large, prospective, cross sectional population study (Bruneck study). *BMJ* 1996; 313:1040-4.

177. *After all, alcohol itself does have a pro-oxidant effect.* Dr. John Folts, personal communication. December 9, 1998

177. *But other studies like the Framingham study...* Schatzkin A, Carter CL, Green SB, et al. Is alcohol consumption related to breast cancer? Results from the Framingham Heart Study. *J Natl Cancer Inst* 1989; 81:31-5.

177. *French, Spanish, and Italian women...* Ellison RC. Here's to your health. Is it now "medically correct" for a physician to prescribe a little wine to lower the risk of heart disease? *Wine Spectator* 1998:35-46.

178. *anthocyanin:* Craig WJ. Phytochemicals: guardians of our health. *J Am Diet Assoc* 1997; 97:S199-S204; Tsuda T, Shiga K, Ohshima K, Kawakishi S, Osawa T. Inhibition of lipid peroxidation and the active oxygen radical scavenging effect of anthocyanin pigments isolated from Phaseolus vulgaris L. *Biochem Pharmacol* 1996; 52:1033-1039.

178. *Catechin:* Hayek T, Fuhrman B, Vaya J, et al. Reduced progression of atherosclerosis in apolipoprotein E-deficient mice following consumption of red wine, or its polyphenols quercetin or catechin, is associated with reduced susceptibility of LDL to oxidation and aggregation. *Arterioscler Thromb Vasc Biol* 1997; 17:2744-52; Lotito SB, Fraga CG. (+)-Catechin prevents human plasma oxidation. *Free Radic Biol Med* 1998; 24:435-41; Valsa AK, Sudheesh S, Vijayalakshmi NR. Effect of catechin on carbohydrate metabolism. *Indian J Biochem Biophys* 1997; 34:406-8; Soleas GJ, Diamandis EP, Goldberg DM. Wine as a biological fluid: history, production, and role in disease prevention. *J Clin Lab Anal* 1997; 11:287-313.

178. *cinnamic acid:* Ekmekcioglu C, Feyertag J, Marktl W. Cinnamic acid

inhibits proliferation and modulates brush border membrane enzyme activities in Caco-2 cells. *Cancer Lett* 1998; 128:137-44.; Mitscher LA, Telikepalli H, McGhee E, Shankel DM. Natural antimutagenic agents. *Mutat Res* 1996; 350:143-52.

178. *ellagic acid:* Barch DH, Rundhaugen LM, Stoner GD, Pillay NS, Rosche WA. Structure-function relationships of the dietary anti-carcinogen ellagic acid. *Carcinogenesis* 1996; 17:265-9; Eaton EA, Walle UK, Lewis AJ, Hudson T, Wilson AA, Walle T. Flavonoids, potent inhibitors of the human P-form phenolsulfotransferase. Potential role in drug metabolism and chemoprevention. *Drug Metab Dispos* 1996; 24:232-7; Stoner GD, Morse MA. Isothiocyanates and plant polyphenols as inhibitors of lung and esophageal cancer. *Cancer Lett* 1997; 114:113-9; Vieira O, Escargueil-Blanc I, Meilhac O, et al. Effect of dietary phenolic compounds on apoptosis of human cultured endothelial cells induced by oxidized LDL. *Br J Pharmacol* 1998; 123:565-73.

178. *These statisticians calculated that heavy drinking accounted for 117 deaths...* Ellison RC. Here's to your health. Is it now "medically correct" for a physician to prescribe a little wine to lower the risk of heart disease? *Wine Spectator* 1998:35-46.

179. *Epicatechin:* Lemaitre D, Vericel E, Polette A, Lagarde M. Effects of fatty acids on human platelet glutathione peroxidase: possible role of oxidative stress. *Biochem Pharmacol* 1997; 53:479-86.

179. *Fisetin:* de Whalley CV, Rankin SM, Hoult JR, Jessup W, Leake DS.Flavonoids inhibit the oxidative modification of low density lipoproteins by macrophages. *Biochem Pharmacol* 1990; 39:1743-50; Fotsis T, Pepper MS, Aktas E, et al. Flavonoids, dietary-derived inhibitors of cell proliferation and in vitro angiogenesis. *Cancer Res* 1997; 57:2916-21; Tzeng SH, Ko WC, Ko FN, Teng CM. Inhibition of platelet aggregation by some flavonoids. *Thromb Res* 1991; 64:91-100.

179. *gentisic acid:* Carlin G, Djursater R, Smedegard G, Gerdin B. Effect of anti-inflammatory drugs on xanthine oxidase and xanthine oxidase induced depolymerization of hyaluronic acid. *Agents Actions* 1985; 16:377-384; Liu J, Smith P. Direct analysis of salicylic acid, salicyl acyl glucuronide, salicyluric acid and gentisic acid in human plasma and using by high-performance liquid chromatography. *J Chromatogr B Biomed Appl* 1996; 675:61-70; Fernandez M, Gracia M, Saenz M. Antibacterial activity of the phenolic acids fractions of Scrophularia frutescens and Scrophularia sambucifolia. *J Ethnopharmacol* 1996; 53:11-14; Tofe A, Bevan J, Fawzi M, et al. Gentistic acid: a new stabilizer for low tin skeletal imaging agents: con-

cise communication. *J Nucl Med* 1980; 21:366-370; Trautmann M, Peskar B, Peskar B. Aspirin-like drugs, ethanol-induced rat gastric injury and mucosal eicosanoid release. *Eur J Pharmacol* 1991; 201:53-58; Personal communication with Dr. Carlos Muller at California State University at Fresno.

180. *Leucocanidol:* Andriambeloson E, Kleschyov AL, Muller B, Beretz A, Stoclet JC, Andriantsitohaina R. Nitric oxide production and endothelium-dependent vasorelaxation induced by wine polyphenols in rat aorta. *Br J Pharmacol* 1997; 120:1053-8; Ferrandiz ML, Alcaraz MJ. Anti-inflammatory activity and inhibition of arachidonic acid metabolism by flavonoids. *Agents Actions* 1991; 32:283-8; Huguet AI, Manez S, Alcaraz MJ. Superoxide scavenging properties of flavonoids in a non-enzymic system. *Z Naturforsch* [C] 1990; 45:19-24.

180. *p-coumaric:* Li P, Wang HZ, Wang XQ, Wu YN. The blocking effect of phenolic acid on N-nitrosomorpholine formation in vitro. *Biomed Environ* Sci 1994; 7:68-78; Sharma RD. Isoflavones and hypercholesterolemia in rats. Lipids 1979; 14:535-9; Sharma RD. Effect of hydroxy acids on hypercholesterolaemia in rats. *Atherosclerosis* 1980; 37:463-8.

180. *polydatin:* Zhang PW, Yu CL, Wang YZ, Luo SF, Sun LS, Li RS. Influence of 3,4,5-trihydroxystibene-3-beta-mono-D-glucoside on vascular endothelial epoprostenol and platelet aggregation. *Chung Kuo Yao Li Hsueh Pao* 1995; 16:265-8.

180. *quercetin:* Chen ZY, Chan PT, Ho KY, Fung KP, Wang J. Antioxidant activity of natural flavonoids is governed by number and location of their aromatic hydroxyl groups. *Chem Phys Lipids* 1996; 79:157-63; Huk I, Brovkovych V, Nanobash Vili J, et al. Bioflavonoid quercetin scavenges superoxide and increases nitric oxide concentration in ischaemia-reperfusion injury: an experimental study. *Br J Surg* 1998; 85:1080-5; Nishino H, Nagao M, Fujiki H, Sugimura T. Role of flavonoids in suppressing the enhancement of phospholipid metabolism by tumor promoters. *Cancer Lett* 1983; 21:1-8; Oguri A, Suda M, Totsuka Y, Sugimura T, Wakabayashi K. Inhibitory effects of antioxidants on formation of heterocyclic amines. *Mutat Res* 1998; 402:237-45; Pace-Asciak C, Hahn S, Diamandis E, Soleas G, Goldberg D. The red wine phenolics transresveratrol and quercetin block human platelet aggregation and eicosanoid synthesis: implications for protection against coronary heart disease. *Clin Chim Acta* 1995; 235:207-219.

180. *Resveratrol:* Chen C, Pace-Asciak C. Vasorelaxing activity of resveratrol and quercetin in isolated reat aorta. *Gen Pharmacol* 1996;

27:363-366; Pace-Asciak C, Hahn S, Diamandis E, Soleas G, Goldberg D. The red wine phenolics trans-resveratrol and quercetin block human platelet aggregation and eicosanoid synthesis: implications for protection against coronary heart disease. *Clin Chim Acta* 1995; 235:207-219; Soleas GJ, Diamandis EP, Goldberg DM. Resveratrol: a molecule whose time has come? And gone? *Clin Biochem* 1997; 30:91-113; Subbaramaiah K, Chung W, Michaluart P, et al. Resveratrol inhibits cyclooxygenase-2 transcription and activity in phorbol ester-treated human mammary epithelial cells. *J Biol Chem* 1998; 273:21875-21882.

180. *First of all, red wine seems to have a greater effect on blood platelets...* Bertelli AA, Giovannini L, Giannessi D, et al. Antiplatelet activity of synthetic and natural resveratrol in red wine. *Int J Tissue React* 1995; 17:1-3; Sauter R, Folts JD, Freedman JE. Purple grape juice inhibits platelet function and increases platelet derived nitric oxide release. *Circulation* 1998; 98:I-585, 3080 (abstract).

181. *salicylic acid:* Muller C, Fugelsang K. Take 2 glasses of wine and see me in the morning. *Lancet* 1994; 343:1428-1429.

182. *tannic acid:* Chung K, Wong T, Wei C, Huang Y, Lin Y. Tannins and human health. *Crit Rev Food Sci Nutr* 1998; 38:421-464; Fitzpatrick D, Hirschfield A, Coffey R. Endothelium-dependent vasorelaxing activity of wine and other grape products. *Am J Physiol* 1993; 265:H774-H778: Kuppusamy U, Das N. protective effects of tannic acid and related natural compounds on Crotalus adamenteus subcutaneous poisoning in mice. *Pharmacol Toxicol* 1993; 72:290-295.

182. *Taxifolin:* Ratty A. Effects of flavonoids on nonenzymatic lipid peroxidation: structure-activity relationship. *Biochem Med Metab Biol* 1988; 39:69-79.

183. *Recent studies have related this to red wine's effect on nitric oxide...* Chen C, Pace-Asciak C. Vasorelaxing activity of resveratrol and quercetin in isolated reat aorta. *Gen Pharmacol* 1996; 27:363-366.

183. *When Dr. Folts from the University of Wisconsin and others, like Dr. Masayoshi Hashimoto...* Hashimoto M, Kim S, Eto M, et al. Acute intake of red wine improves flow-mediated vasodilatation of the brachial artery in men. *Circulation* 1998; 98:1267 (abstract).

183. *Flavonoids play an important role...* Craig WJ. Phytochemicals: guardians of our health. *J Am Diet Assoc* 1997; 97:S199-S204.

183. *His research shows that it is the phytochemicals in red wine...* Sauter R, Folts JD, Freedman JE. Purple grape juice inhibits platelet function and increases platelet derived nitric oxide release. *Circulation* 1998; 98:I-585, 3080 (abstract).

184. *There is even some evidence to show grape juice can lower LDL.* Personal communication with John Folts, University of Wisconsin, January 1999.

184. *Still one more way in which phytochemicals...* Iijima K, Yoshizumi M, Hashimoto M, et al. Red wine polyphenols inhibit proliferation of vascular smooth muscle cells and downregulate expression of cyclin A. *Circulation* 1998; 98:I-599, 3148 (abstract).

Chapter 18: Walk Like an Italian

242. *From the 1960 to the late 1970s obesity in America...* Kuczmarski RJ, Flegal KM, Campbell SM, Johnson CL. Increasing prevalence of overweight among US adults. The National Health and Nutrition Examination Surveys, 1960 to 1991 [see comments]. *JAMA* 1994; 272:205-11.

243. *Nielsen ratings report that hours of TV watching...* Historical Daily Viewing Activity. Nielson Ratings, 1998.

244. *Exercise is helpful not only because it burns calories...* Marcus BH, Albrecht AE, Niaura RS, et al. Exercise enhances the maintenance of smoking cessation in women. *Addict Behav* 1995; 20:87-92.

245. *Research suggests that in most overweight people this is not the case....* Fumento M. *The fat of the land: our health crisis and how overweight Americans can help themselves.* New York: Penguin Books, 1997.

246. *Research has shown that thirty minutes...* Plenary Session XI: Lifestyle Choices and New Pharmacologic Approaches to Prevention of Cardiovascular Disease, American Heart Association Meeting, Dallas, Texas. November 1998.

250. *Dogs are great companions and do wonders...* Anderson WP, Reid CM, Jennings GL. Pet ownership and risk factors for cardiovascular disease. *Med J Aust* 1992; 157:298-301; Beck AM, Meyers NM. Health enhancement and companion animal ownership. *Annu Rev Public Health* 1996; 17:247-57.

Chapter 20: The Mediterranean Alternative Medicine Chest

296. *beta-carotene:* Burton G. Antioxidant action of carotenoids. *J Nutr* 1988:109-111.

297. *benzyl isothiocyanate:* Hecht SS. Chemoprevention by isothiocyanates. *J Cell Biochem* Suppl 1995; 22:195-209; Hamilton SM, Teel RW. Effects of isothiocyanates on cytochrome P-450 1A1 and 1A2 activity and on the mutagenicity of heterocyclic amines. *Anticancer*

Res 1996; 16:3597-602; Hecht SS. Approaches to chemoprevention of lung cancer based on carcinogens in tobacco smoke. *Environ Health Perspect* 1997; 105 Suppl 4:955-63; Hecht SS. Chemoprevention of lung cancer by isothiocyanates. *Adv Exp Med Biol* 1996; 401:1-11; Sugie S, Okamoto K, Okumura A, Tanaka T, Mori H. Inhibitory effects of benzyl thiocyanate and benzyl isothiocyanate on methylazoxymethanol acetate-induced intestinal carcinogenesis in rats. *Carcinogenesis* 1994; 15:1555-60; Wattenberg LW. Inhibition of carcinogenesis by naturally-occurring and synthetic compounds. *Basic Life Sci* 1990; 52:155-66.

297. *beta-ionone:* Jeong TC, Gu HK, Chun YJ, Yun CH, Han SS, Roh JK. Effects of beta-ionone on the expression of cytochrome P450s and NADPH-cytochrome P450 reductase in Sprague Dawley rats. *Chem Biol Interact* 1998; 114:97-107; Jung M, Mo H, Elson CE. Synthesis and biological activity of beta-ionone-derived alcohols for cancer chemoprevention. *Anticancer Res* 1998; 18:189-92; Stratton SP, Schaefer WH, Liebler DC. Isolation and identification of singlet oxygen oxidation products of beta-carotene. *Chem Res Toxicol* 1993; 6:542-7; Wattenberg LW, Loub WD, Lam LK, Speier JL. Dietary constituents altering the responses to chemical carcinogens. *Fed Proc* 1976; 35:1327-31.

297. *carotenoi:* Krinsky NI. Carotenoids: Structure and functions, Proceedings of the Workshop. Potential effects of reducing carotenoid levels on human health, Harvard School of Public Health, January 17, 1996, 1996.

297. *courmarin:* Steinmetz KA, Potter JD. Vegetables, fruits, and cancer. II. Mechanisms. *Cancer Causes and Control* 1991; 2:427-442.

297. *flavonoid:* Baumann J, von Bruchhausen F, Wurm G. Flavonoids and related compounds as inhibition of arachidonic acid peroxidation. *Prostaglandins* 1980; 20:627-39; Craig WJ. Phytochemicals: guardians of our health. *J Am Diet Assoc* 1997; 97:S199-S204. Hertog MG, Feskens EJ, Hollman PC, Katan MB, Kromhout D. Dietary antioxidant flavonoids and risk of coronary heart disease: the Zutphen Elderly Study. *Lancet* 1993; 342:1007-11. Steinmetz KA, Potter JD. Vegetables, fruits, and cancer. II. Mechanisms. *Cancer Causes and Control* 1991; 2:427-442.

298. *glucobrassin:* Bradfield CA, Bjeldanes LF. Modification of carcinogen metabolism by indolylic autolysis products of Brassica oleraceae. *Adv Exp Med Biol* 1991; 289:153-63; McDanell R, McLean AE, Hanley AB, Heaney RK, Fenwick GR. The effect of feeding brassica vegetables and intact glucosinolates on mixed-function-oxidase activity in the livers and intestines of rats. *Food Chem Toxicol* 1989;

27:289-93; Wattenberg LW, Hanley AB, Barany G, Sparnins VL, Lam LK, Fenwick GR. Inhibition of carcinogenesis by some minor dietary constituents. *Princess Takamatsu Symp* 1985; 16:193-203.

298. *hydroxycinnamic acids:* Nardini M, D'Aquino M, Tomassi G, Gentili V, Di Felice M, Scaccini C. Inhibition of human low-density lipoprotein oxidation by caffeic acid and other hydroxycinnamic acid derivatives. *Free Radic Biol Med* 1995; 19:541-52.

298. *indole-3-carbinol:* Bradfield CA, Bjeldanes LF. Modification of carcinogen metabolism by indolylic autolysis products of Brassica oleraceae. *Adv Exp Med Biol* 1991; 289:153-63; Steinmetz KA, Potter JD. Vegetables, fruits, and cancer. II. Mechanisms. *Cancer Causes and Control* 1991; 2:427-442.

298. *isothiocyanates:* Hamilton SM, Teel RW. Effects of isothiocyanates on cytochrome P-450 1A1 and 1A2 activity and on the mutagenicity of heterocyclic amines. *Anticancer Res* 1996; 16:3597-602; Hecht SS. Chemoprevention of lung cancer by isothiocyanates. *Adv Exp Med Biol* 1996; 401:1-11; Hecht SS. Approaches to chemoprevention of lung cancer based on carcinogens in tobacco smoke. *Environ Health Perspect* 1997; 105 Suppl 4:955-63; Hecht SS. Chemoprevention by isothiocyanates. *J Cell Biochem Suppl* 1995; 22:195-209; Huang C, Ma WY, Li J, Hecht SS, Dong Z. Essential role of p53 in phenethyl isothiocyanate-induced apoptosis. *Cancer Res* 1998; 58:4102-6; Steinmetz KA, Potter JD. Vegetables, fruits, and cancer. II. Mechanisms. *Cancer Causes and Control* 1991; 2:427-442.; Sugie S, Okamoto K, Okumura A, Tanaka T, Mori H. Inhibitory effects of benzyl thiocyanate and benzyl isothiocyanate on methylazoxymethanol acetate-induced intestinal carcinogenesis in rats. *Carcinogenesis* 1994; 15:1555-60; Wattenberg LW. Inhibition of carcinogenesis by naturally-occurring and synthetic compounds. *Basic Life Sci* 1990; 52:155-66.

299. *Kaemperol:* Divi RL, Doerge DR. Inhibition of thyroid peroxidase by dietary flavonoids. *Chem Res Toxicol* 1996; 9:16-23; Duarte J, Perez Vizcaino F, Utrilla P, Jimenez J, Tamargo J, Zarzuelo A. Vasodilatory effects of flavonoids in rat aortic smooth muscle. Structure-activity relationships. *Gen Pharmacol* 1993; 24:857-62; Hertog MG, Feskens EJ, Hollman PC, Katan MB, Kromhout D. Dietary antioxidant flavonoids and risk of coronary heart disease: the Zutphen Elderly Study. *Lancet* 1993; 342:1007-11; Nakayama T, Yamada M, Osawa T, Kawakishi S. Suppression of active oxygen-induced cytotoxicity by flavonoids. *Biochem Pharmacol* 1993; 45:265-7; Sathyamoorthy N, Wang TT, Phang JM. Stimulation of pS2 expression by diet-derived

compounds. *Cancer Res* 1994; 54:957-61; Tordera M, Ferrandiz ML, Alcaraz MJ. Influence of anti-inflammatory flavonoids on degranulation and arachidonic acid release in rat neutrophils. *Z Naturforsch* [C] 1994; 49:235-40; Tzeng SH, Ko WC, Ko FN, Teng CM. Inhibition of platelet aggregation by some flavonoids. *Thromb Res* 1991; 64:91-100.

299. *phenethyl isothiocyanate:* Chung FL, Morse MA, Eklind KI. New potential chemopreventive agents for lung carcinogenesis of tobacco- specific nitrosamine. *Cancer Res* 1992; 52:2719s-2722s; Huang C, Ma WY, Li J, Hecht SS, Dong Z. Essential role of p53 in phenethyl isothiocyanate-induced apoptosis. *Cancer Res* 1998; 58:4102-6; Morse MA, Lu J, Gopalakrishnan R, et al. Mechanism of enhancement of esophageal tumorigenesis by 6-phenylhexyl isothiocyanate [published erratum appears in *Cancer Lett* 1997 Jun 3;116(1):117]. *Cancer Lett* 1997; 112:119-25; van Lieshout EM, Peters WH, Jansen JB. Effect of oltipraz, alpha-tocopherol, beta-carotene and phenethylisothiocyanate on rat oesophageal, gastric, colonic and hepatic glutathione, glutathione S-transferase and peroxidase. *Carcinogenesis* 1996; 17:1439-45; Wattenberg L. Inhibition of carcinogenic effects of polycyclic hydrocarbons by benzyl isothiocyanate and related compounds. *J Nat Cancer Insti* 1977; 58:395-398.

299. *protease inhibitors:* Steinmetz KA, Potter JD. Vegetables, fruits, and cancer. II. Mechanisms. *Cancer Causes and Control* 1991; 2:427-442.

299. *quercetin:* Chen ZY, Chan PT, Ho KY, Fung KP, Wang J. Antioxidant activity of natural flavonoids is governed by number and location of their aromatic hydroxyl groups. *Chem Phys Lipids* 1996; 79:157-63; Hertog MG, Feskens EJ, Hollman PC, Katan MB, Kromhout D. Dietary antioxidant flavonoids and risk of coronary heart disease: the Zutphen Elderly Study. *Lancet* 1993; 342:1007-11; Huk I, Brovkovyc/h V, Nanobash Vili J, et al. Bioflavonoid quercetin scavenges superoxide and increases nitric oxide concentration in ischaemia-reperfusion injury: an experimental study. *Br J Surg* 1998; 85:1080-5; Nishino H, Nagao M, Fujiki H, Sugimura T. Role of flavonoids in suppressing the enhancement of phospholipid metabolism by tumor promoters. *Cancer Lett* 1983; 21:1-8; Pace-Asciak C, Hahn S, Diamandis E, Soleas G, Goldberg D. The red wine phenolics trans-resveratrol and quercetin block human platelet aggregation and eicosanoid synthesis: implications for protection against coronary heart disease. *Clin Chim Acta* 1995; 235:207-219.

300. *sulforaphane:* Fahey J, Zhang Y, Talalay P. Broccoli sprouts: an exceptionally rich source of inducers of enzymes that protect against chemical carcinogens. *Proceedings of the National Academy of Sciences* 1997; 94:10367-10372; Nestle M. Broccoli sprouts in cancer prevention. *Nutr Rev* 1998; 56:127-30; Talalay P, Fahey JW, Holtzclaw WD, Prestera T, Zhang Y. Chemoprotection against cancer by phase 2 enzyme induction. *Toxicol Lett* 1995; 82-83:173-9.

300. *terpenoids:* Craig WJ. Phytochemicals: guardians of our health. *J Am Dietetic Assoc* 1997; 97:S199-S204; Haraguchi H, Saito T, Ishikawa H, et al. Antiperoxidative components in Thymus vulgaris. Planta Med 1996; 62:217-21.

Index